Nutrition For The Long Run

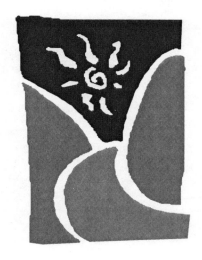

Heidi Smith, BSc, RD
Sport Dietitian

Copies of this and other handbooks can be purchased
in bulk quantities at reduced rates.
Contact Heidi Smith for details.

Heidi Smith, Sport Dietitian
Web: www.heidismithnutrition.com
Email: smithh@uoguelph.ca
Phone: (519) 767 5011
Fax: (519) 821 4007

Cover Photo: Thanks to Peter Fonseca for allowing us to use
his photo from the 1996 Olympic Games Marathon.

National Library of Canada Cataloguing in Publication

Nutrition for the long run : a handbook for runners, walkers, and active individuals / Heidi Smith.

ISBN 1-894933-55-9

1. Runners (Sports)--Nutrition. 2. Exercise.

TX361.R86S63 2003   613.2'024'79642   C2003-905725-9

Table of Contents

Chapter 4: Carbohydrate Loading

Chapter 5: Eating Out at Restaurants

Chapter 6: Sport Supplements

Chapter 7: Recipes

Appendices

Acknowledgements

First and foremost this handbook would not have been possible without the support of Rikki McCarthy and Grace Armstrong from Canada Fit. It was the enthusiasm of Rikki, Grace and their run/walk training groups that inspired the creation of this book.

It is truly amazing how many people have stepped forward to help with the research, revisions and editing of this handbook.

I am indebted to 3 enthusiastic students Sandra Venneri, Suzanne Kaye and Lesley Andrade who volunteered their time during a busy exam period to help pull together each chapter.

My reviewers worked tirelessly under tight time constraints to edit every phrase and punctuation. Thank you to Cyndy McLean, Stephany Cahill, Jasper Blake, Nicole Swerhun, Alix Herber, Stephanie Carter, Mark Neff, Bobby Neff and of course Molly, Mom and Dad for dropping everything to help out in the final hours.

A special thanks to Julie West for her valuable insights and for generously offering her time to review multiple drafts.

And finally, thank you to my husband Aaron and my son Jacob for their support, patience and inspiration.

Introduction

Who Can Benefit From This Handbook

If you are an active individual looking to improve performance and develop lifelong healthy eating habits this handbook can be an invaluable resource. Written by a Sport Dietitian and edited by Physicians, Sport Psychologists, Exercise Physiologists and Athletes, the information is based on sound scientific principles with suggestions that are practical and easy to follow. The chapters were written with runners and walkers in mind, however there is information applicable to anyone who is pursuing an active lifestyle.

How to Use this Handbook

Use the table of contents to guide your way through the topics you find most interesting. The information is organized for quick access to your most pressing questions. There is a wealth of information contained in this small handbook. For best results, try applying the tips and suggestions as small goals over time. For example, one week you may decide to target your hydration, the next week focus on meal timing and so on. You will be amazed how quickly the small goals add up to an overall improved health and performance. Keep this book on hand and use it as a resource during training, before a competition, or any time you are looking for new ideas to improve your nutrition.

I hope this handbook *fuels* your desire to eat right for the long run.

Heidi Smith, Sport Dietitian

1 • Eating for Energy

The importance of nutrition as a foundation for training

The foods you choose on a daily basis have a profound impact on your health, your energy and your performance in sports. The better you fuel your body, the more energy your muscles can store, the faster you recover and therefore the harder you can train. Your "fuel" determines your athletic potential. Food is the foundation of your training!

Food As Fuel

Your body derives energy from 3 main food sources: Carbohydrate, Protein and Fat. In general, carbohydrates are your main fuel for exercise, proteins are the building blocks for muscle and fats provide a concentrated source of energy. Finding the proper balance of these main nutrients is the key to increased energy, longer endurance and faster recovery. To better understand the role of these nutrients, think of your body as a high performance car. Carbohydrates are the "high octane fuel". Carbs are an efficient fuel source that burns clean and fast. You must keep your fuel tank topped up at all times to avoid "running out of gas" therefore you should consume carbohydrates regularly throughout the day. Spend a little extra time and effort to get the high quality "fuel" by choosing complex carbohydrates that are less refined, such as whole wheat breads, pastas and brown rice. Protein is analogous to the engine in your car. You need regular amounts of protein each day to facilitate repairs, in particular repair of muscle after a hard workout. Unlike carbohydrate, protein is not burned as a main fuel therefore you do not need to eat large quantities. Lastly we also need a small amount of high quality fats in the diet to keep everything running smoothly similar to the importance of oil in our car. To complete the analogy, think of water as your coolant. Without adequate water our engines will overheat and we will be forced to cool off at the side of the road.

Achieving the Right Balance

Put into scientific terms, individuals who exercise need a minimum of 55-65% of calories from carbohydrate, 12-15% from protein and 20-25% from fat. Scientific terms are useful for scientists but when serving up your dinner meal, percentages of nutrients may be hard to measure. One method to achieve the right balance is to aim for a dinner plate that is 3/4 carbohydrates (vegetables, grains, fruits) and 1/4 protein (meats, beans, soy, dairy). Even though this looks like 75% carbohydrate, carb sources are bulkier and also contain some protein so that it actually comes out close to the recommended %'s above. Refer to Chapter 3 for more details on meal timing, balance and portions.

Another tool to use is the Canada's Food Guide to Healthy Eating. The Canada's Food Guide was developed for the general public however the principles are very applicable to athletes (Appendix a). The Food Guide advocates choosing whole grain and enriched carbohydrates, emphasizing dark green and orange vegetables and choosing lower fat dairy and leaner protein sources. The recommended food servings will provide approximately 1800-3200 calories with a balance of 55% carbohydrate, 15% protein and less than 30% fat. Some athletes will require additional servings of all food groups to meet their energy requirement. Refer to Appendix d for details on how to get some guidance for setting up a "Specific Eating Plan for You".

Carbohydrate, Glycogen and Endurance

Carbohydrates (carbs) come from any food that is starchy or sweet. Main sources include grains, breads, pastas, fruits, vegetables and to a lesser extent, dairy products. When carbs are consumed they are broken down and stored in the body as glycogen. Glycogen is simply the technical name for stored carbohydrate. Glycogen is stored mainly in the liver (used for blood sugar control) and in our muscles (used as fuel for exercise). In fact, it is one of the only fuels we can burn during anaerobic exercise. Anaerobic exercise can be defined as working at pace where it is difficult to talk without gasping for air. In other words, if you are out of breath or working at a high intensity your main fuel is glycogen. Even in low to moderate intensity exercise such as walking or marathon running glycogen is still the limiting fuel. If you run out of glycogen during a workout you will "hit the wall" and have to stop.

 Think of glycogen as the "wick" in a candle and your fat stores as the wax. If you have no glycogen you cannot sustain a flame and therefore cannot burn energy even with lots of stored fat available. Similar to a candle, our body stores of glycogen (the wick) are very small in comparison to fat stores (the candle wax). Our glycogen stores alone can only sustain high intensity exercise for about 90 minutes. If we used only our fat stores for energy we could theoretically run 4 marathons back to back! Unfortunately fat can only be burned in aerobic conditions and only in the presence of a small amount of glycogen (the wick). So we come back to carbohydrate and glycogen as the limiting factor for endurance exercise. One last point to consider is the ability for glycogen to recover after a workout. If you are exercising for more than 90 minutes you are depleting your glycogen stores. Keep in mind glycogen takes 24-48 hours to fully replenish – even when eating a high carbohydrate diet. Refer to the section "Eating after Exercise" (p.20) for tips on speeding up recovery.

Summary on Glycogen:
It is the storage form of carbohydrate
It is the limiting fuel for endurance exercise
It is needed to burn fat
We have a limited capacity to store it
It recovers slowly
**Therefore athletes need to eat a
high carbohydrate diet.**

Eating Before Exercise

The purpose of a pre-exercise snack is to help maintain your blood sugar until the exercise starts. Carbohydrate from a pre-exercise snack is broken down and absorbed into the blood stream as sugar. The body very closely regulates blood sugar because it is the main fuel used by the brain. If blood sugar drops the brain will trigger a breakdown of glycogen (muscle fuel) and possibly steal essential energy from your muscles. To optimize energy for your workout aim for a small meal or snack 2-3 hours before you exercise. This snack should provide a short-term energy boost to prevent blood sugar from dropping.

The pre-exercise snack does not provide much "fuel" for your workout. Remember from the previous section that it takes 24-48hrs for muscle fuel (glycogen) to store and become available to burn. Therefore during a workout you are not burning your pre-workout snack – you are burn-

> **"During a workout you are not burning your pre-workout snack – you are burning what you ate and stored 24-48 hours earlier"**

ing what you ate and stored 1-2 days earlier. That is why you can get away with a very light snack before a very hard, long workout. For example, some athletes feel best simply drinking a glass of water before exercise first thing in the morning.

The early morning is an exception to the 2-3 hour pre-exercise eating recommendation. Contrary to other times of day, blood sugars can be quite stable upon waking in the morning. If you prefer to exercise before breakfast, on an empty stomach, try a small glass of juice, a piece of toast or even some sport drink 15-30 minutes before exercise. This small amount of easily digested carbohydrate will help raise blood sugar enough to start your exercise feeling energized. Once again, it's not the fuel in your stomach that counts, it's the fuel stored in your muscle and circulating as blood sugar.

The pre-exercise snack can take many forms depending on what time you exercise and what works best for you. Here are some guidelines for choosing food before exercise:

Pre-exercise Eating Guidelines:

1. **Choose foods high in carbohydrate, moderate in fibre, and low in sugar.** Carbohydrate is the main nutrient that keeps your blood sugar stable before exercise. High fibre carbohydrates (>5g fibre per serving) add bulk to your meal and leave you feeling full. Most of the time fullness is a good thing, however 2-3 hrs before exercise you will want food to clear quickly from your stomach. Be cautious with sweet carbohydrates. Sweet carbohydrates have a high glycemic index which means they are absorbed very quickly contributing to a rise and crash in blood sugar levels. A sugar "high" even 30 minutes before exercise may leave you feeling tired and sluggish at the beginning of your workout. Examples of low sugar, moderate fibre carbohydrates: Whole grain products like breads, pitas, low fat, low sugar homemade muffins, cold cereals (low in sugar) or warm cereals like oatmeal, bagels, pasta, potatoes and fruits.

2. **Your pre-exercise meal should contain some protein if eaten more than 2 hours before exercise.** Protein slows the absorption of carbohydrates to help maintain a constant blood sugar level. Choose lower fat protein sources to promote faster digestion. Since protein is digested more slowly than carbohydrate, limit protein intake as you approach the exercise time. (refer to Figure 1) Examples of low fat protein sources: Lean cuts of sandwich meats (eg: turkey or chicken breast, roast beef and ham), light peanut butter, fish (eg: tuna canned in water, varieties like sole or cod), eggs, and low fat dairy or soy products (eg: cheese <20%MF, yogurt 1-2%MF and skim-1% milk).

Figure 1: Composition of Pre-exercise Meals and Snacks

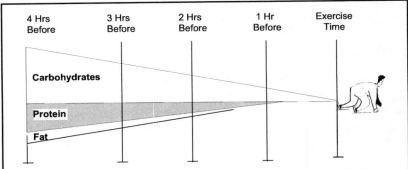

Your pre-meal 3-4 hours before exercise can include carbohydrate with some protein and fat. As you near the time of exercise the size of the meal/snack should decrease and the selection should be primarily carbohydrates with minimal fat and protein.

3. **Choose low fat foods.** Fats slow digestion and may lead to discomfort if eaten too close to exercise. Depending on the size of your pre-exercise meal, limit the total fat intake to about 10-20 grams. (See Chapter 5 for some low fat choices at restaurants) Similar to protein, limit fat as you get closer to your exercise time (Figure 1). <u>Examples of high fat foods to limit</u>: Regular fat cheeses, nuts, sauces (Alfredo), gravies, butter, margarine, fried foods, croissants and baked goods.

4. **Choose foods with which you are familiar and comfortable.** Avoid trying new foods right before a workout. In particular avoid heavily spiced foods such as hot peppers, garlic and onion. These foods can lead to stomach upset and discomfort during exercise. Trial and error will help you determine what's best for YOU!

5. **Maintain adequate fluids throughout the day.** Fluids are a major key to a successful workout. Be sure you are well hydrated before, during and after exercise (see Chapter 2) Drink about 2 cups of fluid 30-60 minutes before you exercise. This will assist stomach emptying during exercise and will help prevent cramping. Avoid drinks that contain

alcohol and caffeine as they can contribute to dehydration. (see Chapter 2 for more details)

Table 1: Pre-Exercise Snack Ideas: Ideally aim for a snack 2-3 hours before exercise, however if you must eat under 2 hours before exercise see sample ideas below.

Time Before Exercise	Composition	Food Ideas
2-4 hours prior	Balanced Meal	Sandwich with low fat toppings, cheese and fruit, trail mix, peanut butter and crackers, soup and salad, pasta with meat sauce, french toast, egg on toast, pizza with low fat cheese(hold the pepperoni)
1-2 hours prior	High Carb, moderate protein, low fat.	Cereal with skim milk, low fat yogourt and fruit, sport bar (<10 grams of protein), yogourt shake (see recipes in Chapter 8)
1 hour prior	High carb, low protein, low fat.	Crackers, sport drink, fruit, toast, 1/2 - 1 bagel with cream cheese, sport bar (<10 grams of protein).

Pre-Exercise Foods to Avoid

1. **High sugar content :** Sugar cereals, candy and candy bars, ice cream and soft drinks
2. **High in dietary Fibre:** Beans (any kind), prunes, gassy vegetables (eg: broccoli, onions, cauliflower and brussel sprouts).
3. **High in fat:** Full fat dairy products (eg: cheese, ice cream and full fat milks), chocolate and chocolate bars, high fat meats (eg: chicken wings and sausages), anything deep fried such as potato chips.
4. **Fast Foods:** Cheeseburgers, hotdogs, tacos, wings, greasy pizzas, french fries and anything else deep fried.

Eating During Exercise: Increasing Endurance

The most effective way to spare glycogen stores and increase endurance is to consume carbohydrates during exercise lasting longer than 90 minutes. Most of us have enough glycogen to "keep our flame burning" for about 1.5 hours of continuous high intensity exercise. However, after 90 minutes without a source of carbohydrate from food or drink, complete exhaustion is just around the corner. Complete exhaustion is also known as "bonking" or "hitting the wall" - A very unpleasant experience where you are physically unable to continue exercising. To avoid "The Wall" aim to consume 0.7-1g of carbohydrate per kg of body weight per hour during exercise.[1] This works out to about 30-60 grams of carbohydrate per hour of exercise You should start consuming carbohydrate after the first 60-90 minutes.

Carbohydrate is the only fuel your body needs during exercise therefore seek food and drink sources low in protein or fat. Popular sources include sport drinks, bars and gels. See Chapter 6 for a comparison of different products. Supplements are convenient and usually designed for easy digestion however, good old fashioned food can produce equal results. See Table 2 for some common foods used during exercise

Guidelines when choosing food to consume during exercise:

1. Look for carbohydrate foods that are low in fibre (<5g fibre per serving). Fibre is essential in your regular diet, however it is too slow to digest during exercise.
2. For high intensity exercise (>60% of your max), avoid fats and protein since they will also slow digestion (<5g protein or fat per serving).
3. Consider how convenient the food is to carry and eat while exercising.
4. Be sure to consume a minimum of 2-4 cups of fluid with any solid food you choose. Consuming a food without adequate fluid can cause stomach upset and indigestion.
5. Consume foods in small amounts over the hour rather than all at once.
6. Always try a food several times during training to be sure it works for you before trying it in a race.

Table 2: Common Foods Used During Exercise
(Keep in mind recommendation of 40-60 grams of carbohydrate per hour of exercise)

	Serving Size (g)	Cals (kcal)	Carb (g)	Sodium (mg)	Fibre (g)	Protein (g)	Fat (g)
Bagel – plain (110g)	1	302	59	587	2.5	11.5	2
Banana – medium	1	108	28	1.2	2.8	1.2	0.6
Raisins	1/4 cup	124	33	5	1.6	1.3	0.2
Dried apricots	1/4 cup	79	20	3	3	1.2	0.2
Arrowroots	4 (20 g)	88	14	74	0.04	1.6	2.8
Baked potato	1 (172 g)	188	43.5	14	4	4.0	0.4
Saltines	10	118	20	356	0.8	3.0	2.8
Pretzels (low fat)	12	100	23	400	0.9	3.0	2.1
Graham Crackers	4 (28g)	119	21	185	0.9	2.0	2.8
Fat Free Fig Bars	4	260	62	244	1.6	2.0	0.4
Low fat granola bar	1 (26 g)	110	20	40	1.2	1.1	2.5
Homemade Sport Drink: water with 5 tsp of honey, 1/8 tsp salt	500ml	100	25	250	0	0	0

Three Easy Steps For A Workout Eating Plan
Here is an example of how to use a combination of foods, fluids and supplements during a 3 hour workout.

1. Calculate your carbohydrate needs based on 0.7-1g carb/kg/hour. eg: A 70 kg athlete = 50-70g carb per hour after the first hour
2. Choose a combination of food and/or fluid that appeals to you. eg: Pretzels, Gatorade sport drink, Powerbar sport bar
3. Using the tables of carbohydrate values provided, plan out the quantities needed and the timing. Remember, for best absorption it is best to spread your carbohydrate consumption over the hour.

1st Hour	500-750ml water
2nd Hour	500ml Gatorade (28g carb): 12 Pretzels (23g carb): Eat 3 every 15 minutes
3rd Hour	1 Powerbar (45g carb): Eat 1/4 every 15 minutes, 250ml Gatorade (14g carb), 250 ml water

Eating After Exercise: Faster Recovery

After a hard workout your glycogen stores will be depleted, you may be dehydrated and your muscles will need some repair and rebuilding time. The body needs 24-48 hours to fully replenish glycogen stores after an endurance workout. 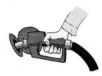 If you are working out every other day, recovery may not be a problem. Your regular high carbohydrate diet will help to restore your "fuel tank" of glycogen in due time. Many athletes however, train every day and sometimes several times per day. In these cases fast recovery can be critical to keep pace with a busy training schedule. One of the most effective ways to increase recovery time is to eat immediately after a workout. There

> **"If you provide the right fuel soon after exercise you can double the speed of glycogen recovery."**

is a "recovery window" of 2 hours following a workout. During this 2 hour time your muscles are in overdrive trying to repair and replenish. A snack within 15-30 minutes post exercise provides the fastest recovery. If you can provide the right fuel soon after exercise you can double the speed of glycogen recovery. This can be an incredible performance enhancing tool because you can maximize your energy stores in a shorter amount of time. That means you'll be ready for your next workout sooner. Follow these tips to make the best use of your "recovery window":

Eating Tips for Faster Recovery From Exercise:

1. **Consume a high carbohydrate, moderate protein snack** immediately after your workout preferably within 15-30 minutes. See Table 3 for some ideas.
2. **The post workout snack should contain a minimum of 50 grams of carbohydrate** along with a source of protein (7-15 grams of protein should be adequate). A small amount of protein may help the muscle repair faster.[3] Larger amounts of

carbohydrate are needed because this is the fuel that has been burned. Simply consuming a normal high carb training diet composed of frequent small meals and snacks every 2-3 hours will help achieve glycogen recovery. See Chapter 3 for tips on meal timing and balance to ensure constant recovery throughout your day.

3. **Drink enough water** during your workouts to maintain your weight. Maintaining your weight ensures you drank enough to balance sweat losses. Staying adequately hydrated will help your circulation to carry lactic acid and waste products away from the muscle. Lactic acid is one of the culprits causing muscle soreness post exercise. Appendix f has a weight log to help you track your level of hydration before and after exercise. Chapter 2 also details tips for adequate hydration.

4. **Take at least one recovery day per week.** Adequate recovery time can be as essential as adequate training time. Allow at least one full day for your muscles to completely re-fuel and repair.

Table 3: Post Workout Snack Ideas

Snack	Cals (cal)	Carbs (g)	Protein (g)
2 cups of chocolate milk (with 1% milk or soymilk)	340	56	17
2 cups of chocolate milk (made with skim milk powder)*	278	50	18
1 litre (4 cups of 6-8% carbohydrate sport drink)	224	56	0
1 cup milk (or soymilk), 1-1/4 cup cereal (eg: Vector)	275	53	13
Banana and low fat yogourt (175ml)	250	48	13
Peanut butter and jam sandwich	350	50	12
300ml Sunny Orange Shake*	278	51	11
1 c Trail mix made with dried fruit and cereal *	280	40	15

* See Chapter 7 for recipes

2 • Hydration

The Importance of Hydration

Water is the foundation of performance both in exercise and in daily life. It is perhaps the most underestimated nutrient when it comes to performance enhancing capacity. Muscle is made up of 75% water and even a 3% loss in water can cause a 10% reduction in strength and an 8% reduction in speed![1] Many athletes are chronically dehydrated without even knowing it. The problem is that our thirst mechanism does not "kick in" until approximately 3% dehydration. That means by the time you are thirsty you may have already lost 10% of your performance! Athletes and active individuals must "think to drink" in order to prevent dehydration. We cannot rely on thirst to guide our fluid consumption.

> **"By the time you are thirsty you may have already lost 10% of your performance"**

Why do we need fluids?

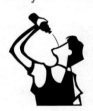

The body is made up of 65-75% water. It is an essential daily nutrient needed for almost every major bodily function. During exercise, water forms the liquid portion of your blood which helps carry oxygen and nutrients to working muscles while taking away wastes to be eliminated in the urine. It is also the foundation for sweat production to regulate body temperature during exercise. Blood pressure and heart rate are affected by hydration along with organ cushioning and joint lubrication. Water is needed for the storage of fuel into the muscle.

How Does Dehydration Reduce Performance?

As mentioned previously, a 3% dehydration (4.5 pounds in a 150 pound athlete) can reduce muscle performance by 10%.[1] Table 4 outlines the different stages of dehydration. There are many mechanisms by which dehydration affects performance. In particular, as water becomes scarce, the body loses its ability to sweat and regulate body temperature. If you compare this situation to a low coolant level in a car – you risk "overheating" leading to heat exhaustion if you don't drink enough fluids. If you rarely sweat during a workout this could be a sign

> **"A loss of just 2 lbs of fluid can increase heart rate by 8 beats/minute"**

you are dehydrated! Increased sweat production is actually a sign of better fitness. As your fitness level improves you will start to sweat sooner, sweat volume will increase and you will lose less electrolytes (eg: salt and potassium) in your sweat. Therefore, it is of critical importance to continue increasing your fluid consumption as you increase your training.

Table:4 Stages of Dehydration and Performance Effects

% Body Weight Loss	Weight Loss Based on 120-180lb athlete	Effect on Health and Performance
2%	2.5-3.5 lbs	Reduced ability to control temperature, increased heart rate.
3%	3.5-5.5 lbs	Decreased muscle endurance. 10% Decline in performance.
4-6%	4.5-11lbs	Decreased hand-eye coordination, decreased muscle strength and endurance.
>6%	>7bs	Increased respiration rate, decreased blood volume, nausea, and confusion.
>10%	>12 lbs	Heat stroke and exhaustion. A serious life threatening condition.

Adapted from the Sport Nutrition Advisory Council of Canada. [5]

Heart rate is another major mechanism affected by hydration. A loss of just 2 lbs of fluid can increase heart rate by 8 beats/minute. If you've ever checked your heart rate during a workout, a difference of 8 beats per minute over an hour workout can make a big difference in your level of fatigue. A study published in the Journal of Sports Science showed that dehydrated exercisers had significantly reduced endurance. Poor hydrators worked out for 25% less time than those who drank water before and during workouts.[2] Other unpleasant side effects of dehydration include: decreased concentration, cramping, nausea, and headaches.

How much do we need?

During the day: Adults need to drink at least 8-10 cups (1 cup = 8oz = 250ml) per day of non-caffeinated fluids in addition to drinking during and after exercise.

During exercise: Aim to consume 2-4 cups (500ml-1Litre) of fluid per hour of exercise. For maximal absorption, fluids should be sipped frequently throughout rather than gulping large amounts infrequently. For example, 1/4 cup (50-60mL) every 5-10 minutes. Drinks should be dilute with no more than 6-8% carbohydrates. (Gatorade: 6%, eload: 6%, Powerade: 8%, Juice: 10%, Pop: 11%). Drinks such as juice and pop are too concentrated and therefore can draw water into the stomach instead of being absorbed out of the stomach. Consuming a carbohydrate content over 8% can result in stomach cramping, bloating and nausea. Chapter 6 outlines tips for choosing sport drinks and shows a comparison of different products.

After Exercise: Weigh yourself before and after exercise to determine how much fluid you lost. To replenish fluids lost during exercise you need to drink 3 cups (750 ml) of fluid for every pound lost. It was once thought that 2 cups per pound was adequate however more recent research indicates 3 cups are needed to regain the pound.[7] That can add up to a LOT of fluid if you don't drink enough

> **"Weight lost during a workout is water loss, not body fat loss"**

during exercise. Even a modest 2 lbs of water loss equates to 1.5 litres of water you need to drink after the exercise to rehydrate! Prevention is the best strategy. Drink enough during your workout to maintain your weight. Weight lost during a workout is water loss not body fat loss. Body fat loss occurs over weeks and months, not in the time frame of a workout.

Use the hydration weight log in Appendix f to determine how much you need to drink to maintain your weight during exercise. Factors such as weather, temperature, sweat rate, clothing worn, pre-exercise hydration state and choice of drink, will all affect the rate at which you lose fluids during a workout. The weight log chart will help you develop strategies for different conditions and different workouts.

What about Caffinated Beverages?

Caffeine is a central nervous system stimulant, meaning it increases heart rate, alertness, blood pressure and gastro-intestinal rate. Beverages that contain caffeine such as colas, coffee, or tea may stimulate fluid loss and promote dehydra-tion.[3] More recent research indicates caffeine is not a strong diuretic. The bottom line is that every person is affected by caffeine differently. The best way to prevent the ill effects of caffeine is to use it in moderation. Aim for a maximum of 2-3 caffinated beverages per day. In addition, ensure you are drinking your base of 8-10 cups of non-caffinated fluids.

Can Caffeine Increase Endurance?

The short answer is - yes. However there are many things to consider before adding a pre-workout pot of coffee. The research indicates that high levels of caffeine can increase endurance when taken 1-2 hours before an endurance workout.[6] Interestingly, coffee itself was not as effective. There appears to be something in the coffee that nullifies the benefit of the caffeine for endurance. The only way to get the endurance effect is to take a caffeine pill equivalent to the caffeine amount in 6-8 cups of coffee!

There is also speculation that even small amounts of caffeine may stimulate the brain and alter your perception of how hard you are working, making the exercise seem easier. Some athletes enjoy a cup of coffee or a cola 1-2 hours before a workout. Many claim they feel more energized and eager to get started. Another interesting note is that caffeine will not stimulate water loss during exercise. Exercise overrides the normal diuretic effect of the caffeine. If you wish to experiment with caffeine, always do so in training first. Take into consideration that caffeine is a stimulant and it can cause irritability, stomach cramping and even diarrhoea. Stimulants also have withdrawal symptoms therefore if you consume caffeine regularly and stop suddenly you can expect headaches, fatigue and even flu-like symptoms. Therefore avoid changing your caffeine habits right before a competition.

Caffeine is also a regulated substance by the International Olympic Committee. If you are a competitive athlete, the equivalent of 6-8 cups of coffee in one sitting is enough to disqualify you with a urine test.

What about Beer and Alcohol?

Some research indicates that 1 drink a day can reduce risk for several chronic diseases. Alcohol can be a relaxing and enjoyable part of a meal or social event. Unfortunately, the effect on athletic performance is not as positive. You should abstain from alcohol 2-3 days before any major competition to ensure adequate hydration and storage of muscle glycogen. Alcohol is a diuretic meaning that it can promote dehydration. In addition, alcohol interferes with the speed of glycogen storage and recovery. If you recall from previous sections, glycogen (stored carbohydrate) is the limiting fuel for exercise and therefore critical before competitions. Contrary to popular belief, beer is not a good source of carbohydrate and it can in fact slow down your storage of carbohydrate if taken after

> **"Contrary to popular belief, beer is not a good source of carbohydrate"**

exercise. In summary, enjoy your alcohol in moderation. Save it for days when fast recovery and hydration are not a priority.

Practical Tips: Overcoming Obstacles

How can I remember to drink enough?
- Try carrying a water bottle with you everywhere you go.
- Try drinking a tall glass of water with your meals and snacks.
- Try filling a 1.5 L bottle and drink it throughout the day (6 cups)

Is there any way to help reduce the number of trips to the bathroom?
- At first, you might find you need to use the bathroom several times per hour! Fear not, your body will get used to the higher amount of fluids you are drinking if you stick with it. Your kidneys will eventually adjust to this higher amount and your visits to the bathroom will decrease. Expect at least 2-3 weeks to adjust.
- A sport drink with sodium and electrolytes may decrease urine output during exercise. NB: "eload" sport drink has one of the highest electrolyte levels. (See Chapter 6 for sport drink comparisons)

Is it really worth carrying that extra weight of water during my runs?
- The short answer is YES! Water is one of the most powerful sport supplements. You can easily become dehydrated even on a cool day. Carrying and drinking water to avoid dehydration could mean a 10% improvement in your muscle performance. During long runs, if you can't carry all your fluids try planting water bottles along your running route. Get accustomed to wearing a water belt or "camelback".

During a running race, how can I be sure I'm drinking enough from those little cups?
- When drinking, equate an ounce with a gulp – so 8 to 10 adult gulps are approximately an 8-ounce serving.[4] Even better, measure your own "gulp capacity". Take a 1 cup (8oz) measure full of water and count how many gulps it takes for

you to finish the whole cup. During a race you will then know exactly how much you are getting from the little cups. Another race tip – when drinking from paper race cups, squeeze off the opening of the cup so you can seal your mouth over the opening and suck out the water. This will help avoid swallowing air and choking on the water.

What if fluid before/during activity makes me feel sick?
- If you get cramps or a "sloshy" feeling when you drink you may have been dehydrated at the start of your exercise. If you are well hydrated before exercise starts, your stomach may absorb the fluids more easily. Try to drink at least 8 cups during the day including 2 cups in the hour before exercise. This will help you stomach absorb the fluids faster during exercise.

Is it possible to drink TOO much?
- Yes. This is rare but it does happen, especially in prolonged (> 2 hrs) high intensity exercise in hot weather. When you drink too much plain water it dilutes the sodium in your blood and it may cause headaches, nausea, dizziness, poor performance, and high blood pressure. To prevent over-hydration, do not drink more than 1 L/hr of plain water during exercise. Take a sport drink if you need more fluids. With exercise > 1 hr, use a sports drink that contains sodium (eg. eload, Gatorade, Allsport…). Refer to Table 7 for sodium contents of different sport drinks. Consult a Sport Dietitian before resorting to salt tablets.

3 • Achieving a Healthy Weight

3

What Is A Healthy Weight?

What is a healthy weight? Every person would have a different answer to this question. Healthy, physically fit bodies come in all shapes and sizes. Not even the popular "Body Mass Index" (BMI) charts can accurately predict the ideal weight for a physically active individual. BMI uses a ratio of your weight to height as a predictor of health risk. Weight and height are only 2 of many factors used to define a healthy weight. Other factors include: body fat, muscle mass, bone structure, bone density, gender, age, heredity, disease risk, eating preferences, sport demands and social pressures.

> **"Healthy, physically fit bodies come in all shapes and sizes."**

When choosing a goal weight it is important to be realistic about the change your own body is capable of maintaining. Rather than start with a goal of achieving an arbitrary "number" on the scale, why not focus on developing the healthy habits that will lead to a healthy weight. It is a way of giving your own body the power to reach it's top potential.

Some key habits affecting weight include: proper meal timing and portions, adequate hydration, balanced nutrition and a balanced exercise routine. Changing habits does not happen overnight and therefore finding the best weight for your body will take time. If you give yourself at least a one year commitment to the pursuit of healthy eating and exercise habits you will be well on your way to achieving your ideal weight. The following sections will provide you with some guidance on developing healthy eating habits to achieve a healthy weight.

Optimal Meal Timing

What if one simple eating strategy could help you to: achieve an optimal weight, increase energy, reduce body fat, avoid overeating, reduce cravings for carbohydrate, reduce cholesterol, improve recovery and increase endurance? The suggestion sounds almost too good to be true. However, all of these health benefits are associated with the simple tool of maintaining blood glucose levels.

Blood glucose is a measure of sugars circulating in the blood. When we digest food, sugars are broken down and absorbed into the blood stream. These sugars are essential for normal brain function and survival. Therefore the body strives to maintain a stable blood glucose level (also called blood sugar level) throughout the day. Stable blood sugars are achieved through a combination of glucose from food, hormone regulation and stored energy sources (glycogen and fat). Figure 2 illustrates how daily blood sugars can fluctuate. Symptoms of low blood sugar are also noted to the left of the graph.

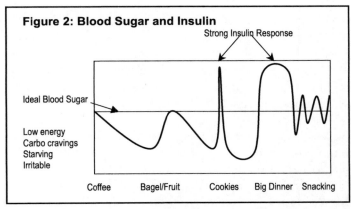

Figure 2: Blood Sugar and Insulin

Notice how skipping breakfast can cause blood sugars to drop resulting in low energy, cravings for carbohydrate and a propensity to overeat in the evening. The afternoon bagel and fruit provide a short boost in energy however due to the lack in protein, blood sugar levels fall soon after and create another carbo craving. The following section "Achieving The Right Balance" explains the importance of combining protein and carbohydrate for stable blood sugars. The cookies raise blood sugar rapidly triggering a strong insulin response. Insulin is a hormone that brings blood sugars down. However, as shown in figure 2, a strong insulin response can sometimes overshoot and leave you feeling low soon after a snack or meal.

The most common symptom of poor meal timing is overeating at dinner. If you are "starving" when you start a meal you will be more likely to overeat. Excess calories from this large meal along with high levels of insulin will promote the storage of body fat. Some people may even experience carb cravings and urges to snack in the evening. This may be a result of an insulin "over shoot" from the large dinner. And to think, all of this could have been prevented by eating breakfast and planning balanced small meals and snacks.

Figure 3 demonstrates this ideal meal timing and balance. Blood sugar levels are kept stable by small meals and snacks every 3-4 hours.

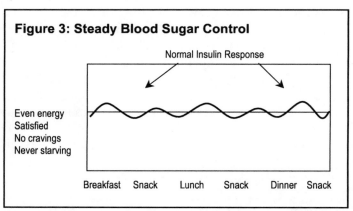

Figure 3: Steady Blood Sugar Control

Energy is steady, while cravings and hunger are satisfied. Less insulin is required to regulate blood sugars. Once again insulin is a "storage hormone" that promotes body fat storage and cholesterol production. The effect of lower insulin levels may be one of the reasons why frequent small meals has been shown to reduce cholesterol by as much as 10% in individuals with high cholesterol.[2] In addition, lower insulin and smaller meals will promote body fat burning by making it easier to eat less and create a calorie deficit.

Achieving The Right Balance

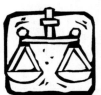

Focus on making balanced food choices each time that you eat. A balanced snack is one that contains carbohydrate and a source of protein. The carbohydrate provides you with some quick energy and the protein helps to make that energy last longer. For example, a piece of fruit (carbohydrate) will provide you with energy for only 1-2 hours. If you combine the fruit with a piece of cheese (protein) you may stay satisfied for 3-4 hours. The combination helps to maintain a slow rise and fall in blood sugars.

Satisfying snacks should also be low in sugar with a source of fibre. The sugar raises blood glucose rapidly triggering a strong insulin response and possibly leaving you feeling low even 30 minutes after the snack. Conversely, fibre slows the rise in blood glucose and therefore helps to extend the energy of the snack. For example whole wheat bread is a better carbohydrate choice than white bread. See Appendix b for a list of complex carbohydrates and lower fat protein choices. As a quick reference, carbohydrates are mainly foods that are "starchy or sweet". Protein foods are generally more savoury. Some popular combinations listed in Appendix b include: crackers and cheese, peanut butter and celery, yogourt and fruit, soy nuts and raisins.

Soy Nuts – A Tasty Source of Protein

Soy nuts are soy beans that have been cooked and roasted. They come in different flavours including: barbeque, salted, unsalted and even honey coated (more suitable as a dessert than a snack). They are a great source of fibre and have about double the protein of nuts with half the fat. Some varieties however are oil roasted which will put fat content at par with nuts. Look for dry roasted varieties in the health food section or bulk food section of your grocery store. If a food label is available – look for varieties less than 10g of fat per 1/4 cup serving.

How Can Snacking Help Me Lose Weight?

Adding balanced snacks between your meals can help you lose weight if (and only if) you reduce the size of your main meals. In other words you will be spreading out your food intake throughout the day and avoiding any large meals. The ultimate goal for weight loss is to reduce calorie intake. Therefore choose small balanced snacks that are under 250 calories. Refer to Appendix b for some ideas. Your hunger will be satisfied, your cravings blunted and therefore it will be easier to eat less total calories in the day. It is very different from being on a low calorie diet and trying to ignore your hunger. Food is your friend, rather than your enemy.

Should I Snack If I'm Trying to Gain Muscle or Maintain Weight?

Yes! If you are trying to gain muscle, snacking can help provide the much needed fuel and protein to build muscle. If you tend to lose weight easily, add in extra snacks whenever you can throughout your day. Higher calorie snacks such as trail mix, dried fruit, chocolate milk and juices can help to provide the necessary calories without excess bulk.

How Much Should I Eat?

Your best guide for quantities and portions is to listen to your hunger. Once you have achieved a steady energy pattern by choosing frequent small meals, you will be able to "trust" your hunger. Hunger pangs will indicate that your blood sugar is dropping and it's time for a meal or snack. If you ignore your hunger OR are too busy to stop and eat, you run the risk of hitting a low blood sugar and consequently overeating at your next meal. This comes back to the importance of eating every 3-4 hours so that you stay within a moderate hunger range.

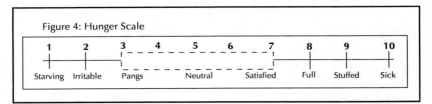

Figure 4: Hunger Scale

Figure 4 outlines a tool you can use to measure your hunger. Ideally you should aim to start eating soon after noticing hunger pangs (between 3-4) and stop eating just when you are satisfied (6-7) before you feel full or stuffed (8-9). Many people eat simply because "it is lunch-time" or finish their plate "because it's there" rather than tuning into their body's internal cues. You will be more likely to overeat if you wait until you are irritable or starving (1-2). In other words, if you start eating at a hunger rating of 1-2 you will probably eat quickly and end up at a rating of 9-10 (stuffed or sick). Try some of these practical tips when monitoring your level of hunger and fullness.

Tips For Eating The Right Amount Of Food:
1. <u>Keep a journal of food intake.</u> Writing down what you eat will make you more aware of portions and meal timing. Try writing down everything you eat for a minimum of 3-4 days. Refer to Appendix e for a sample food record and food recording tips.

2. <u>Eat slowly</u> during a meal so that you have time to recognize your level of fullness. It is best to stop eating when you are "satisfied", before you are "full". This may mean leaving food on your plate even if you *could* eat it. By waiting 10-15 minutes you may find you feel just right, instead of full. Overall, a good rule to give yourself 20 minutes to eat your meal and evaluate your fullness.

3. <u>Try leaving food on your plate.</u> Even if it is just 1 bite, try to overcome the habit of eating just to clean your plate. An interesting study looked at 2 groups of women. One group was instructed to eat normally, the other was told to always leave at least 1 bite (or more) on their plate. The group who left food on their plate appeared to stop eating earlier and consequently lost an average of 10 pounds over a 1 year period. Those last bites really do add up!

4. <u>The standing test.</u> If you are in the midst of your meal and feeling out of touch with your level of fullness – stand up and go for a short walk. Taking a break to go to the bathroom, get something from the kitchen, change the radio station etc… This short break may help you re-focus on how full you really feel.

5. <u>Try to minimize distractions at meal/snack time.</u> Our lives are full of distractions. It can sometimes be very difficult to stay aware of our own internal cues such as hunger and stress. A study compared men who consumed a meal while watching tv, listening to a mystery on the radio or eating with neither. Those who had the distraction of tv or radio tended to eat on average 300 calories more.

6. <u>Watch out for deep sighs.</u> If you find yourself sitting back, loosening your belt, or feeling the need to take a deep breath – you are probably approaching "stuffed".

**Sometimes YOU SHOULD EAT
Even In The Absence Of Hunger:**

- *Not hungry for breakfast?* Try to eat breakfast within 1 hour of waking up. This boost of energy will also boost your metabolism. You may even notice you are more hungry after eating breakfast than if you hadn't eaten at all! This is actually a good sign that you have jump started your metabolism. You are off to a good start of eating more during the day (when you need it) and less at night.

- *Not hungry with your morning coffee?* When you are drinking coffee or caffinated beverages the caffeine can act as an appetite suppressant. Some people actually use coffee to help 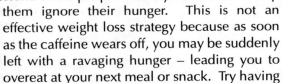 them ignore their hunger. This is not an effective weight loss strategy because as soon as the caffeine wears off, you may be suddenly left with a ravaging hunger – leading you to overeat at your next meal or snack. Try having a balanced snack mid morning with a bottle of water instead of a coffee. This will satisfy your hunger early, help you stay hydrated and provide your body with "real" energy instead of the "fake" energy from caffeine.

- Not hungry after exercise? Exercise can be an appetite suppressant. If you are trying to increase your speed of recovery it is best to eat within 15-30 minutes following exercise even if you are not hungry. If you are not exercising every day, recovery is less of an issue and you can wait until your hunger re-surfaces.

- Not hungry when you are stressed or distracted? A busy lifestyle sometimes makes it difficult to stop and eat at the proper times. Try to develop a regular schedule of meals and snacks every 3-4 hours to help train your hunger. Make eating a priority even when you are stressed or very busy. Use a snack as a much needed break in between meals. A snack can take less than 5 minutes which is time well spent when you consider the energy boost and clarity of mind it can provide.

**Sometimes YOU SHOULD NOT EAT
Even If You Do Feel Hungry:**

• *Hungry right after a large dinner?* If you refer back to Figure 2 (p.32) you will notice that "hunger" after a large meal may be due to a high insulin response and a subsequent crash in blood sugars. If your craving is strong to eat something, try to keep it small and satisfying (eg: balance of protein and carbohydrate, low in sugars). This will help to get blood sugars and hunger back on track.

• *Hungry when you are stressed?* Often people turn to food when they are coping with stress. If you have eaten within 2-3 hours it is probably not a true hunger. Look for other non-food ways to cope with the stress such as going for a walk or run, stretching, talking with a confidante, taking a bath etc...

• *Hungry when you are dehydrated?* Sometimes thirst can be mistaken for hunger, especially in hot or dry environments. If you are "hungry" soon after a meal/snack try having a cold glass of water. You may find this satisfies the urge to eat.

Weight Loss Woes

Many people start an exercise program with a goal of shedding some extra pounds. In particular, most would like to lose pounds of body fat while retaining their muscle. This can be a frustrating pursuit if you are using the scale to measure your success. It is a well-known fact that exercise can promote increases in muscle and decreases in fat. In many cases the increased weight of new muscle balances out the losses of fat weight. After several months of exercise you may find yourself at the same weight despite a rigorous workout routine and careful eating habits. Some may view this as a failure and can lose motivation to continue exercising. One question you may want to ask your self is:

"Why Do I Want To Lose Weight?"

To Reduce Risk of Disease? You can significantly reduce blood pressure, improve insulin sensitivity and reduce cholesterol without shedding a single pound. Simply an increase in exercise with a reduction waist circumference (smaller belt size) can improve all of the health indictors mentioned without losing "weight".[1] Furthermore, a modest 10% weight loss in a year (A 200 pound person losing 1-2 pounds per month = 20lbs/year) can significantly reduce risk for chronic diseases such as diabetes, cancer and heart disease.

To Look and Feel Better? Exercise has the incredible capacity to increase energy, improve breathing, reduce stress, and tone muscles - making you look and feel better even in the absence of weight loss.

To Perform Better In Your Sport? Carrying less weight can have a performance enhancing effect for some sports. On the other hand inadequate calorie consumption can slow down your recovery, reduce your endurance and leave you feeling drained. To improve performance you are better off focusing on optimal fuelling rather than cutting calories to lose weight.

Tips to Avoid Weight Loss Woes

1. Put your scale away. Weight alone is not an accurate indicator of health for athletes. Scale weight does not take into account your ratio of muscle to body fat. For example: according to the BMI (Body mass index) chart, a man who is 5'8" and 190 lbs is over weight. However, this man may be very fit, with a high bone density and strong muscles.

2. Find other motivators besides weight to help you measure success. Set small achievable goals such as: increasing weights in the gym, faster running times, longer endurance, walking a steep set of stairs without getting out of breath, reducing a belt notch, fitting more comfortably in your clothing, increased energy, better sleeping, ...be creative and track your goals weekly or monthly on paper. Small measurable goals will give you something concrete to motivate you in your quest for lower body fat. If you would still like to use a measurement to track your body fat loss there are a few measures you an use as a more accurate alternative to the scale. Waist circumference, Skinfold measurements and Bioeletcrical impedance analysis (BIA) are 3 ways to track potential changes in body fat. Ask your local gym or fitness centre if they provide any of these services.

3. Weight fluctuates with your state of hydration. Just 1 bottle of water (500ml) weighs 1 pound. If you are dehydrated or even retaining water your scale will not give you an accurate picture of changes in body fat. Therefore if you are looking to lose 1-2 pounds per week the scale can be very frustrating. Yet another reason to put the scale away.

4. Give yourself time. What's the rush. Wouldn't you rather lose the body fat slowly, preserve your muscle and keep it off for longer? Many people make the mistake of hurrying the "transformation" by starving themselves or over-exercising thereby burning away muscle, exhausting themselves and

eventually regaining the weight. There are no proven short cuts. The next section describes some sensible guidelines to achieve a lower body fat while maintaining optimal health.

Burning Body Fat

Body fat is an important fuel source not only during exercise but also during every moment of your day. At rest you are deriving about 60% of your energy from body fat with the remaining 40% coming from carbohydrate (stored as glycogen). The amount of fat stored on your body is dictated by your energy balance. If calories in (food) = calories out (exercise) your body fat will remain the same. You may still be burning body fat during your workout but it will be restored by the calories you eat.

> **"The key to losing body fat is to create an energy deficit."**
> *Calories In < Calories Out*

The key to losing body fat is to create an energy deficit. It comes down to simple math you must either eat less, burn more or a combination of the two. It is important to make changes in your calorie intake slowly and modestly. You should always provide enough calories to maintain your "basal metabolism" which is the base amount of calories for you to breathe, pump your heart and support life. To calculate your estimated basal metabolic rate (BMR) refer to Figure 4.

Figure 4: Estimating Basal Metabolic Rate

Basal Metabolic Rate (BMR) is an estimate of the calories your body requires to fuel your basic life support systems. This value does not take into account calories needed for daily activity, exercise or stress (see figure 5).

Men (calories per day)
18-30 yrs: $(0.0630 \times \text{weight(kg)} + 2.8957) \times 240$
31-60 yrs: $(0.0484 \times \text{weight(kg)} + 3.6534) \times 240$

Women (calories per day)
18-30 yrs: $(0.0621 \times \text{weight(kg)} + 2.0357) \times 240$
31-60 yrs: $(0.0342 \times \text{weight(kg)} + 3.5377) \times 240$

Adapted From: Harrison's Principles of Internal Medicine, 1998

If your calorie balance begins to approach your BMR, your body may go into "starvation mode" and begin to protect your fat stores while burning away muscle. The exact opposite of your goal! This survival mechanism prevents starvation by burning away tissues that use up calories. Muscle uses lots of calories whereas fat does not. Therefore in a starvation state, the body cleverly gets rid of the "calorie expensive" muscle while protecting the "calorie rich" fat. The way to lose body fat is eat less than you burn (or burn more than you eat) without approaching your BMR. For example: Jane is a 45 year old woman, 163 pounds (74 kg), running 2-3 times per week. Using Figure 4, her BMR is estimated at about 1450 calories per day. Her energy expenditure is estimated at about 2200 per day. (see Figure 5) To burn body fat at this moderate activity level she must eat between 1500 and 2200 calories per day.

Figure 5: Estimating Energy Expenditure	
Energy Expenditure = BMR x Activity factor.	
	Activity Factor
Low (sedentary)	1.3
Medium(some regular exercise)	1.5
High (regular exercise or physical job)	1.7
Very High (athlete)	Consult a Sport Dietitian

Keep in mind the equations provided in figures 4 and 5 are crude estimates. They are meant to provide "ballpark" figures for calorie needs to help prevent under-eating. Counting calories is not a long term solution for maintaining a healthy weight or a healthy outlook on eating. One of the best ways to eat the right amount for a lean body weight is to eat frequent small meals and snacks in amounts to satisfy your hunger. See earlier sections for a more detailed description of optimal timing, portions and balance.

What Burns More Calories: Walking or Running?

The age-old argument between walkers and runners is whether you burn more calories walking a mile or running a mile. The truth is – you burn the same amount of calories to travel a mile, regardless of speed. The only significant difference is that the runners will finish the mile faster. If you have only 30 minutes to exercise and you want to lose body fat, running will burn the most calories. In contrast – if you are not in a hurry you can walk the same distance as you would have run and you will burn the same calories.

What is Better for Reducing Body Fat: Walking or Running?

If you recall from Chapter 1, fat is an aerobic fuel meaning you need adequate oxygen to burn body fat. In contrast, glycogen is an anaerobic fuel meaning it can be burned even in the absence of oxygen. Walkers may argue that walking is more aerobic therefore the main source of energy they are burning is fat! They dare not break into a jog and risk becoming anaerobic thereby switching to glycogen as the main fuel. The runners will argue they are working harder so they burn more calories. Both groups are correct as demonstrated by the pie graphs that follow.

Fuel Source During Exercise

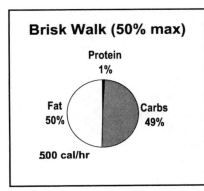

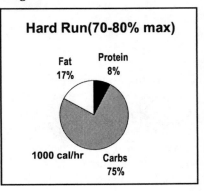

Walkers derive a higher percentage of their fuel from body fat (50% for walkers vs 17% for runners) however, runners burn more calories in a shorter time (500 calories per hour vs 1000

calories per hour). Even though the high intensity runner burns less fat during the workout – they will burn more calories per hour and create a bigger calorie deficit. Once again, it comes back to simple math. At the end of the day the person who creates the biggest calorie deficit (calories out > calories in) will lose the most body fat.

The bottom line: To reduce your body fat % it doesn't matter if you walk or run. Nor does it matter how much fat you burn during your workout. Fat loss boils down to - burning more calories than you eat.

Is it Possible to Lose Body Fat Without Losing Weight?

Yes! It is quite common for people to begin an exercise program, increase muscle mass and not notice changes in scale weight. This simply means the person has reached an energy balance. The amount of food they are eating is providing the energy and building blocks to make muscle, while still creating a deficit to promote the burning of fat. Some may perceive the stable weight as an indication the exercise program is "not working". However for many people, weight loss is not really the ultimate goal. Improved strength, fitness and an attractive body shape is often the goal. Therefore the best guide once again is to eat frequent meals and snacks according to your hunger. If you are at a healthy weight your hunger will increase to match your activity level therefore helping you to build muscle, burn fat and maintain weight.

4 • Carbohydrate Loading

What is Carbohydrate Loading?

Carbohydrate loading (carbo-loading) is the combination of eating high carbohydrate foods and tapering exercise before an endurance event. The goal of carbo-loading is to maximize the amount of carbohydrate stored in the muscle. It always includes a carbohydrate loading stage, which is sometimes preceded by a carbohydrate depletion stage, though the depletion stage has not been shown to be necessary for success.[1]

In exercise lasting longer than 90 minutes, carbohydrate loading can significantly increase time to exhaustion (aka "Hitting the wall"). Carbohydrates are stored in the muscle and liver in the form of **glycogen**. Glycogen is the limiting fuel for endurance events such as marathons, half-marathons, cycling and triathalons.[2] See Chapter 1 for more details on glycogen and performance.

Which Athletes Can Benefit From Carb-Loading?

As mentioned above, carb-loading can help any athlete improve endurance in events lasting longer than 90 minutes. This would apply to the more obvious endurance events such as marathons however also can apply to multi-event weekends for sports such as swimming, hockey, soccer, tennis, basketball, field hockey etc... When multiple exercise times add up to more than 90 minutes glycogen can become depleted. Carbohydrate loading is not recommended for one time events lasting less than 90 minutes such as a 5km or 10km running race. Every gram of glycogen is stored with 3 grams of water. Therefore, the extra stored weight of glycogen can be detrimental in some short duration events.

Good Sources of Carbohydrates

Top sources of carbohydrate include breads, cereals, fruits, vegetables, legumes and even milk products. Anything sweet or starchy will contain carbohydrates. Focus on complex carbohydrates, which are found in whole grains, beans, fresh fruit and vegetables. A high source of carbohydrate can be considered >15g of carb per serving.

Table 5: Carbohydrate Content of Some Common Foods

Food	Carb (g)	Food	Carb (g)
1 medium bagel	45	1 cup rice	45
1 cup beans	45	Powerbar	45
1 cup pasta	30	1 cup fruit yogurt	40
2 cups cooked veggies	20	1 cup cooked peas or corn	30
8 saltine crackers	16	1 cup fruit juice	30
1 cup sports drink	15	1 potato	30
1 cup milk	12	1 granola bar	15

How Much Carbohydrate Do I Need?

When you look down at your plate, 3/4 should be made up of grains, fruits and veggies and 1/4 should be protein. For a more precise amount, you can calculate your carbohydrate requirement: 6-8 grams of carbs per kg body weight.[3] This means roughly 300-500 grams of carbohydrate for a 140-150 pound athlete training 1-2 hours per day. This carbohydrate level would translate into about 8-10 servings of grains, 4-5 servings of fruits, 4-5 servings of vegetables and 3-4 servings of milk products. Check the Canada's Food Guide (Appendix a) for serving amounts. Following this plan will give you about 60-65% of your calories from carbohydrates (assuming a 2000-3000 calorie diet). Appendix c shows a sample 60-65%, 2500 calorie diet. If you are looking for a specific eating plan tailored to your needs refer to Appendix d.

Sample Race Nutrition Countdown

7 Days Before The Race

You should begin to taper your workouts, by roughly 50% every second day.[4] The taper is important to allow your muscles time to maximize glycogen stores. You should also be tapering your calorie intake to adjust for less exercise. A rough guideline is to cut back by 250-500 calories per day once the taper begins. To adjust your calories cut back on extra fats such as butter/ margarine, salad dressings, chips (See calorie and fat values below) Save your calories for the much needed carbs.

Some examples of ways to save on calories from fat:

1 Tbs	Butter, margarine, olive oil, vegetable oil	10g fat	90 calories
2 Tbs	Regular salad dressing	10g fat	100 calories
1 Tbs	Mayonnaise	12g fat	110 calories
1	Small bag of chips	25g fat	300 calories
1	Med order of fries	20g fat	400 calories

6-5 Days Before The Race

Continue adjusting your intake and concentrating on a variety of complex carbohydrates. Use your hunger as a guide for reducing your intake. Be sure to eat enough by eating frequently (every 2-4 hours), but be careful not to stuff yourself. It is very important not to miss meals and snacks.

4 Days To Go

These last 4 days are the most critical for topping up glycogen stores. Include bread and grains with meals and use fruit and fruit juices in your snacks. Be sure to still include some protein with meals and snacks but watch carefully for fat content. If you are reading food labels look for meals under 10-15 grams of fat, and snacks under 5 grams of fat.

3 Days To Go

Your training should be at a bare minimum by now. You may be starting to feel heavy and sluggish, but don't panic! This is a good sign. The extra weight means that your body is successfully loading up on carbohydrates. Every gram of carbohydrate is stored with 3-5 grams of water![5] You can expect to gain 2-8 pounds of water/glycogen weight (not fat weight!). It may feel heavy now but you will be thankful to have carried the extra fuel when you hit the halfway mark in your race.

2 Days Left
Fluids, Fluids, Fluids. Your body is using lots of fluids to pack in the glycogen so try to drink enough water to dilute your urine to a near clear yellow. You should expect to visit the washroom at least every 2-3 hours, if not more often. A general guideline is to consume a minimum of 2.5-4 litres each day before the race (10-16 cups). If you are having trouble getting in that much plain water you can dilute juices or use a sport drink, which provide carbohydrate as well. It is also a good idea to munch on some salty foods to maximize your electrolytes. Some high salt items include: pretzels, crackers, soups, cheese, cottage cheese, pickles and lightly salting foods.

The Day Before
You should take a rest from your training today. Continue with frequent small meals, but do not overstuff yourself as you want to have speedy digestion today. Think of it as "grazing" on complex carbohydrates and drinking 1-2 cups of fluids per hour to stay hydrated. Avoid alcohol today as well as any foods that may upset your stomach.[6] Some gassy and irritating foods to avoid include: broccoli, cabbage, beans, spicy foods, and fried foods. Don't try any new foods today, stick to the old faithful meals you know and love. Glycogen takes at least 24 hours to store in the muscle so by dinner-time you should be fully topped up. This also means dinner should not be huge. Stick to a small low fat, high carbohydrate meal such as pasta and tomato sauce, turkey sub, rice dish….

Race Day
Eat a light breakfast the day of the race. It's too late to store glycogen BUT your body will use the breakfast meal to keep your blood sugars stable. Stick to your usual breakfast, don't try

anything new. Most people do best with a light breakfast 2-3 hours before the race. A sample meal could include a toasted bagel with peanut butter, banana and glass of juice OR a bowl of your favorite cereal (hold the sugar, not too much fibre) and some water or juice. Try to drink consistently throughout the morning before your race (1-2 cups per hour) and be sure to consume at least 2 cups in the hour prior to your race. If you get hungry you can nibble on some easily digested foods such as 1/2 sport bar or saltine crackers[6]. Another option is to drink a sport drink such as Gatorade to keep your blood sugars stable before the race. The last thing to do is warm-up, stretch and relax – You have a full fuel tank to conquer the challenge ahead of you!

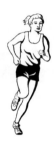

4 • Carbohydrate Loading

5 • Eating Out At Restaurants

Making the Best Choices

With a full schedule jam packed with work, family, friends and training, you may find yourself relying on restaurant foods to get you through a busy week. Race weekends or competitions requiring travel will also present the challenge of finding low fat, high carbohydrate choices while eating on the road. This chapter will provide you with some comparisons of different restaurants and some practical tips for making the best choices.

Eating out can be the result of a rushed schedule, lack of desire to cook or simply an opportunity to socialize with friends and family. It's a treat to have others cook for you and there's no clean up afterwards! Some athletes will even confess that part of their drive to exercise is to have the room to indulge on decadent foods from time to time. Decadent indeed - restaurant portions are notorious for being unnecessarily large and high in fat. You may find you feel tired and sluggish after a restaurant meal. If you refer back to Chapter 3 (Figure 2) you will recall the effect of large meals on blood sugar and insulin. A good guideline is to limit eating out to 1 time per week. If you are eating out more than 1 time per week use the following tips and restaurant comparisons to make the best choices.

Tips for Eating at Restaurants

1. When looking at the menus, look for key words that describe low fat or high fat foods. Low fat food adjectives normally include grilled, steamed, broiled, boiled, marinara, poached and baked. High fat foods typically are those that are prepared by frying, sautéing, or include au gratin, alfredo, cream or butter.

2. While eating in Italian restaurants, order pasta with red/tomato/marinara type sauces. Thick crust pizzas will be higher in calories however they are also packed with valuable carbohydrates. Ask for extra bread, but be aware of keeping butter intake to a minimum. Avoid cheesy lasagnes, cream sauces and chicken/eggplant parmesan due to their high fat content.

3. At Asian restaurants, order steamed rice rather than fried, choose dishes with vegetables and low fat protein sources like chicken. Lo mein and stir-fried dishes are better choices than deep-fried choices like egg rolls or sweet and sour dishes. Sushi is an excellent high carbohydrate, low fat choice. Just to be safe on competition weekends, order versions made with cooked seafood only. Request foods to be free of MSG (mono-sodium glutamate), a food additive that may trigger headaches or stomach upset.

4. Roadhouse or pub-style restaurants usually offer a soup, salad and bread option. Ask for dressings and butter on the side so you can control portions. Club sandwiches can be an excellent choice. You can reduce the fat content by asking for the toppings on the side and the bacon crispy (or omit it). Stay away from high fat foods such as wings, fish and chips, coleslaw, Caesar salad, nachos, chicken pot pie, chicken fingers and fries.

5. In Mexican restaurants, order pot beans instead of refried beans, and ask for baked tortillas instead of deep-fried shells. Limit use of sour cream and guacamole; instead, use extra salsa.

Tips for Choosing Fast Foods

1. Refer to Table 6 for a comparison of different fast food choices. Most establishments will provide you with the nutrition information if requested. Plan meals that are less than 20 grams of fat and snacks that are less than 10 grams of fat.

2. An excellent alternative to the typical high fat burger and fries meal is a grilled chicken sandwich. Look for varieties that are not breaded since these are usually deep fried.

3. To improve hydration, order beverages that are caffeine free such as juice, water, clear pop, caffeine free tea or milk.

4. If eating within a day of competition try to refrain from the pressure to order "super size" or "biggie". Some fast food operations will try to sell you bigger portions for only pennies more. From a strictly financial perspective it is tempting. However before a competition quick digestion can be critical so aim for frequent smaller meals rather than a "super size" feast.

5. Controlling portion size can also be a way to offset the extra calories if necessary. For example, order the small size french fries or split a higher fat item.

6. Add carbohydrates with baked potatoes, salads, juice, milk and/or frozen yogurt.

7. Sub Shops offer an excellent variety of high carb, low fat options. Choose your toppings wisely, the fats from cheese, sauces and mayos can quickly add up.

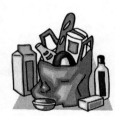 Lastly, heading to the grocery store before, during or after a trip can provide you with healthy, high carbohydrate foods at a fraction of the cost of dining out. You can pick up fresh fruits, dried fruit, chopped vegetables, bagels, bread, soynuts, trail mix, granola bars, low fat cheese and yogourt. Also stock up on fluids such as water, juices and sport drinks. Many grocery stores also have ready-made foods like roast chicken, submarines and salad bars. These choices offer healthy, high carbohydrate foods at affordable prices.

Table 6: A Comparison of Restaurant Choices

Lower Fat Choices (Meals< 20g, Snacks <5g fat)

McDonalds www.mcdonalds.ca/en/ourmenu/index.asp

Lower Fat Choices	Cal	Fat	Carb	Pro
Hamburger	246	7.9	31	12
Cheeseburger	295	12	32	15
Chicken McNuggets(6)	293	17	18	18
Egg McMuffin	292	12	29	17
Mc Veggie Burger	359	7	50	24
Chicken McWrap	377	10	52	21
Mandarin California Greens w/ Fat Free Raspberry Vinaigrette Dressing & Trail Mix	424	19	55	9.5
Large Frozen Yogurt Cone-Chocolate	299	6.5	51	8.7
Fruit 'n Yogurt Parfait	156	2.5	31	4.1

Higher Fat CHOICES to LIMIT Meals > 20g, Snacks >5g fat

Choices to Limit	Cal	Fat	Carb	Pro
Big Mac	541	30	44	24
Quarter Pounder w/Cheese	534	30	37	30
Big Extra	662	40	47	28
Sausage McMuffin w/Egg	467	26	35	22
French Fries (Large)	519	24	70	5
Big Breakfast	636	36	49	27
Triple Thick Shake - Vanilla, Medium	726	15	134	14
Baked Chocolate Chip Cookie	180	9	24	3
Large McFlurry - Smarties	713	20	119	14

Lower Fat Choices (Meals< 20g, Snacks <5g fat)

Dairy Queen www.dairyqueen.com/content/brand_menu/nutrition/nutchartlimited.pdf

Lower Fat Choices	Cal	Fat	Carb	Pro
Medium Vanilla Cone	330	9	53	8
M&M's Treatzza Pizza (1/4 pizza)	190	7	29	3
Fudge Bar (no sugar added)	50	0	13	4
Beef Sandwich	300	9	37	16

Higher Fat CHOICES to LIMIT Meals > 20g, Snacks >5g fat

Choices to Limit	Cal	Fat	Carb	Pro
Brownie Earthquake	740	27	112	10
Blizzards (Medium)	640-950	23-36	97-143	12-17
Banana Split	510	12	96	8
Super Dog	580	37	39	20

Lower Fat Choices (Meals< 20g, Snacks <5g fat)

Subway   www.subway.com/subwayroot/MenuNutrition

Lower Fat Choices	Cal	Fat	Carb	Pro
Steak and Cheese	390	14	48	24
Subway Melt	410	15	47	25
Honey Mustard Ham*	310	5	52	18
Chipotle Southwest Turkey Bacon*	410	16	48	22
Sweet Onion Chicken Teriyaki *	380	5	59	26
*Ham, *Roast Beef, *Roast Chicken Breast, *Subway Club, *Turkey Breast, *Turkey Breast + *Ham, *Veggie Delite	230-320	3-5	40-50	9-25
Lite Mayo (1 Tbs)	45	5	1	0

Higher Fat CHOICES to LIMIT Meals > 20g, Snacks >5g fat

Choices to Limit	Cal	Fat	Carb	Pro
BMT	480	24	47	23
Meatball	540	26	53	23
Cold Cut Trio	440	21	47	21
Tuna	450	22	46	20
Golden Broccoli Cheese Soup	180	12	12	6
Toppings like mayonnaise, sub sauce (1 Tbs)	110	12	0	0
Horseradish sauce	90	10	1	0

Values are for 6" subs—double values for 12"   * Indicates cheese NOT included

Lower Fat Choices (Meals< 20g, Snacks <5g fat)

Swiss Chalet   www.swisschalet.ca/ourmenu/nutritionals.pdf

Lower Fat Choices	Cal	Fat	Carb	Pro
1/4 Chicken, White, No Skin	225	8	0	40
1/4 Chicken, Dark, No Skin	232	10	0	35
Grilled Santa Fe Chicken Sandwich	523	15	59	39
Veggie Burger	404	11	51	25
Stir Fries (Veggie/ Chicken)	218-372	3-7	42-40	5-39
SantaFe Grilled Chicken Salad, no dressing	274	9	17	31
Chicken Soup	97	2	11	9

Higher Fat CHOICES to LIMIT Meals > 20g, Snacks >5g fat

Choices to Limit	Cal	Fat	Carb	Pro
Golden Grilled Chicken Caesar Salad	832	53	41	49
Warm Chicken Salad Amandine	868	60	42	40
Baked Garlic Cheese Loaf	696	29	84	26
Club Wrap	621	24	58	44
Big Beef Burger	637	30	48	43
Wings-Medium	914	53	50	63
French Fries	470	25	53	8
Ribs (Regular)	753	55	5	59

Lower Fat Choices (Meals< 20g, Snacks <5g fat)

Burger King   www.burgerking.com/Food/Nutrition/InteractiveWizard/index.html

Lower Fat Choices	Cal	Fat	Carb	Pro
Hamburger	315	13	31	16
Chili	200	9	19	14
Chicken Tenders (6)	250	14	15	16
Garden Salad	25	0	5	1
Chunky Chicken Salad	220	7	5	35
BK Veggie Burger	335	10	47	13

Higher Fat CHOICES to LIMIT Meals > 20g, Snacks >5g fat

Choices to Limit	Cal	Fat	Carb	Pro
Whopper	770	45	51	34
King Supreme Sandwich	559	34	32	30
BK Fish Fillet	446	22	44	18
Chicken Sandwich	565	29	52	25
French Fries (Medium)	360	18	46	4
Vanilla Milkshake (Medium)	720	41	73	15

Lower Fat Choices (Meals< 20g, Snacks <5g fat)

Wendy's   www.wendys.com/CanadianNutrition.pdf

Lower Fat Choices	Cal	Fat	Carb	Pro
Junior Hamburger	311	12	33	15
Junior Cheeseburger	355	16	37	17
Grilled Chicken Sandwich	302	7	36	24
Chicken Breast Fillet Sandwich	396	15	44	24
Spicy Chicken Sandwich	397	13	45	24
Baked Potato, Plain or with Sour Cream	310-370	0-6	73	7
Chili (large)	300	9	31	25
Small Frosty	330	8	56	8
Mandarin Salad without dressing	345	16	30	25
Fat Free French	87	0.1	21	0.4
Reduced Fat Ranch	111	8.6	6.4	1.9

Higher Fat CHOICES to LIMIT Meals > 20g, Snacks >5g fat

Choices to Limit	Cal	Fat	Carb	Pro
Big Bacon Classic	570	29	46	34
Classic Single (With Everything)	410	19	37	24
French Fries (small)	313	13	45	4
French Fries (Biggie)	440	19	63	5
Taco Supreme Salad with chips	676	34	60	32
Broccoli & Cheese Potato	580	22	81	18
Chicken BLT Salad with Dressing	657	44	30	35
Spring Mix Salad with Dressing	509	42	13	27
Mandarin Salad with dressing*	596	34	50	26
Side Caesar Salad with Dressing*	292	23	8.5	12.5
Ranch Dressing	266	26	5.6	1.7

* Fats are higher than recommended however most fats are unsaturated (healthy fats)

Lower Fat Choices (Meals< 20g, Snacks <5g fat)

Tim Horton's www.timhortons.com/english/english.html

Lower Fat Choices	Cal	Fat	Carb	Pro
All Bagels	<320	<4	<58	10
Harvest Turkey Breast, Fireside Roast Beef, Albacore Tuna Salad, & Chunky Chicken Salad Sandwiches	370-470	9-18	50	21-27
Chili	244	9	24	17
All Soups (not cream)	110-150	2-3	15-25	3-5
Cream Soups	235-245	9-11	26-31	6-9
Lowfat Muffins	280	2	60-65	5-7

Higher Fat CHOICES to LIMIT Meals > 20g, Snacks >5g fat

Choices to Limit	Cal	Fat	Carb	Pro
Cookies (per cookie)	135-155	5-9	20	2
Tea Biscuits	230-480	7-20	38-70	5-7
Garden Vegetable Sandwich	451	23	51	10
Cherry Cheese Danish	380	23	33	7
Cream Cheese, light-regular	110-140	3-13	3	2
Regular Muffins	310-410	10-20	50-65	5-8

Lower Fat Choices (Meals< 20g, Snacks <5g fat)

Harvey's http://www.harveys.ca/eng/site.php

Lower Fat Choices	Cal	Fat	Carb	Pro
Veggie Burger	331	9.2	41	21
Grilled Chicken	299	5.2	35	28
Crispy Chicken	380	10	48	23
Fish Sandwich	352	10	49	16
Original Hamburger	357	18	32	18
Chicken Nuggets	172	9.4	11	11
Garden Salad	121	5.9	11	6.5
Vegetable Soup	118	1.7	25	2.5

Higher Fat CHOICES to LIMIT Meals > 20g, Snacks >5g fat

Choices to Limit	Cal	Fat	Carb	Pro
French Fries (Large)	474	25	57	6.2
Onion Rings (Regular)	286	20	23	4
Onion Rings (Large)	431	30	34	6
Poutine	700	40	67	20
Ultra Burger with Cheese	457	2	34	31
Blueberry Muffin	376	19	62	6.1
Vanilla Milkshake	370	9.9	59	11

Food values for table 6 were sourced from the websites of each respective food estbalishment, where available. For a complete listing of foods offered at these establishments refer to each company website.

6 • Sport Supplements

Using Sport Supplements

There are a vast array of sport supplements on the market today. The tables which follow summarize just a few of the different products available. Supplements can be useful during training for quick, convenient and easily digestible energy. However, avoid becoming a supplement "junkie". If you rely on bars, drinks and gels morning, noon and night you are not optimally fueling your body. Supplements are not meant to replace real food. Appropriately named, they should "supplement" a healthy, balanced diet. Even though some contain vitamins and minerals they should not be considered whole foods. Whole foods contain a complex mix of nutrients and active ingredients that cannot be perfectly duplicated. Make whole foods the foundation of your diet and enjoy the convenience of supplements sparingly.

> **"Avoid becoming a supplement "junkie"- Appropriately named, they should supplement a balanced diet"**

6

Sport Drinks

Sport drinks should be regarded as the sport supplement with the greatest potential to enhance performance in a wide variety of sporting situations. It is well known that proper hydration, adequate electrolytes and a source of carbohydrate can increase endurance and improve performance. Sport drinks are likely to promote better fluid intake than water because they generally taste better. They also may increase retention of fluid consumed post-exercise by reducing urine losses. Not all sport drinks are created equal. Some are more difficult to absorb, some have lower levels of electrolytes and some are not optimally balanced for absorption during exercise. Use the following tips to choose your sport drinks wisely:

Tips for Choosing Sport Drinks

1. Always try out a supplement during training at least 2 weeks BEFORE a competition. Find out what works for YOU.

2. During exercise carbohydrate is the most easily digested energy source. The harder you exercise, the harder it is to digest anything except simple carbohydrate. For example: During a brisk walk or hike you should be able to easily digest a drink or food which contains a mix of protein, fat and carbohydrate. As you increase your intensity toward a fast paced run (over 60% of your max) you will only be able to digest carbohydrate. Carbohydrate foods, sport drinks and gels are your best bet for higher intensity exercise. If you experience cramping or stomach upset with sport supplements look for a sport drink with no more than 6-8% carbohydrate and avoid drinks with Fructose, Sucralose and/or High fructose corn syrup. (see Table 7)

3. Remember that some drinks/bars are designed specifically for recovery and should be taken AFTER exercise. If taken during, their high protein, fat and % carbohydrate content could cause stomach upset.

4. Real food can also be used as a "sport supplement". Refer to Table 2 in Chapter 1 for some inexpensive and effective alternatives to bars, gels and drinks. Remember to always try these foods in training before a competition.

Table 7: Sport Drink Product Comparison
Based on 16 fl oz (500ml) serving

Name	Cals	Carb (g)	Type of Carb	Carb %	Pro (g)	Fat (g)	Sodium (mg)	Potassium (mg)
Eload	110	27	Dextrose, sucrose	5.4	0	0	370	96.5
Gatorade	125	28	Sucrose, glucose, fructose	5.6	0	0	220	60
All Sport	140	38	High fructose corn syrup	8.0	0	-	110	100
Cytomax	100	20	Maltodextrins, fructose, amylopetcin	4.0	0	0	100	150
PowerBar Perform	120	32	Glucose, fructose, maltodextrins	4.8	0	0	165	52
PowerAde	174	44	High fructose corn syrup, maltodextrins	8.8	0	0.5	110	100
Revenge Sport	90	23	Maltodextrin, dextrose, amylopetcin, fructose	4.6	0	0.5	100	147
Ultima	53	13	Maltodextrins	1.6	0	0	16	31
G Push Endurance	190	48	Maltodextrin, galactose, fructose	4.8	< 1	0	170	40
MET-Rx	240	64	Sucrose	12.8	0	0	30	-
Hydra Fuel	99	25	Dextrose, fructose, maltodextrin	5.0	0	0	37.5	74
White Lightning	225	28	High fructose corn syrup, maltodextrin, sucralose	5.6	29	-	211	160
Sport Drinks with protein (not appropriate for use during high intensity exercise)								
Accelerade	187	35	Sucrose, fructose, maltodextrin	7.0	9	1.0	253	85
EnduroxR4	360	71	Glucose, Fructose	14.2	17	1	293	160
Metabolol Endurance	200	24	Fructose, dextrose, maltodextrin	6.4	19	7	280	400
Mass Recovery	338	53	Maltodextrin, sucralose	10.6	31	-	303	143
MET-Rx – Chocolate	250	22	Maltodextrins	3.8	38	2.5	380	1200

- Dash indicates value unknown

Energy Bars

There seem to be more energy bars on the market than ever before. Walking into a supplement store can be a mind-boggling experience. Keep in mind there is nothing magical about "energy bars". They do not provide MORE energy than real food and they tend to be quite expensive. They are however fast, easy and portable. Use them sparingly and choose wisely using the following tips...

Tips for Choosing Energy Bars:

1. If using the bar DURING exercise you should choose a bar with lower protein, fibre and fat. Protein, fibre and fat are slow to digest and can cause stomach upset during high intensity exercise.

2. If using a bar as a snack between meals, choose one with 7-15 grams of protein to ensure lasting energy. Avoid bars high in sugar or fat when using them as a snack. Keep in mind calorie intake if your goal is to lose body fat. Some bars exceed 300 calories and may be too much for an athlete trying to economize on calories.

3. Bars can be used to supplement protein intake, HOWEVER they do not contain all of the nutrients found in whole protein sources such as meats and dairy products. Bars also may contain a high level of sugar and hydrogenated oils. If you are using protein bars more than 3 times per week to supplement protein intake seek advice from a registered sport dietitian to find some better long term solutions.

4. If using a bar to recover from a workout, be sure the bar contains a minimum of 30 grams of carbohydrate and 7 grams of protein. After exercise, carbohydrate is the most important fuel to replenish. Ideally a minimum of 50 grams of carbohydrate is preferable. In particular, carbohydrate from "sugars" will travel quickly to the muscle to help restore glycogen.

Table 8: Energy Bar Product Comparison

Note: different flavours have different nutritional values

	Serving Size (g)	Calories	Carb (g)	Sugar (g)	Fiber (g)	Protein (g)	Fat (g)
PowerBar Harvest	65	260	45	22	2	7	5
Clif's LUNA Bar	48	170	29	17	3	10	2
Gatorade Bar	65	260	46	20	2	15	5
Balance Bar	50	200	22	18	1	14	6
Genisoy ProteinBar	61.5	220	33	27	1	14	4
Power Bar Performance	65	230	45	20	3	9	2.5
Zone Perfect Bar	50	210	22	13	0	16	7
Promax Bar	75	290	38	34	1	20	6
Ironman Hi Energy	56.8	230	26	23	1	16	8
Soy Sensation Bars	50	180	22	11	5	15	6
Bio-Protein Bar	81	300	39	32	1	21	7
Extreme Body Bar	85	320	18	10	1	34	7
Meso-Tech Bar	85	340	44	29	0	25	7
BuzBar	50	200	18	-	-	18	6
Nitro-Tech Bar	88	290	31	2	2	35	7
Protein Plus Bar	78	270	36	19	2	24	5
Methoxy-Pro Protein Bar	80	280	15	7	1	30	7
WARPbar	50	180	31	-	-	8	3.5
Tri-o-plex	118	327	36	9	5	30	7
Atkins Nutritional Advantage Bar	60	230	20	0	2	20	10
Clif Bar	68	240	43	21	5	10	4

- Dash indicates value unknown

Sport Gels

Gels are a concentrated source of carbohydrate. The benefit of gels is their compact portability and ease to eat while exercising. A draw back of gels is their high concentration of carbohydrate which can be difficult to digest while exercising. Use the following recommendations when choosing gels...

Tips for Using Gels

1. Try using gels in training to see how they affect your stomach.
2. A gel pack should be taken with 500ml of fluid in order to maintain a 6-8% concentration of carbohydrate. If a gel is taken too quickly without enough water it may not dissolve or absorb properly. Water may be drawn into the stomach from surrounding tissues causing a "sloshing" feeling, improper water absorption, cramping and stomach upset.
3. Ideally, a gel should be taken in small amounts over the course of 45 min-1 hour. This will allow you time to drink fluids along with the gel to ensure proper absorption. For example: try taking a "squirt" of your gel every 15 minutes along with water or sport drink – rather than all at once.
4. You can buy gel "flasks" where you premix your gels with some water to make it easier to take in small amounts. The flask attaches to a belt or fits in your water carrier for easy access.

Table 9: Sport Gel Product Comparison

	Serving (g)	Calories	Carbs (g)	% CHO	Sodium (mg)	Potass-ium (mg)	Protein (g)	Fat (g)
Power Gel	41	120	28	68%	50	40	0	1.5
Clif Shot	32	100	24	75%	50	50	0	0
GU	32	100	25	78%	20	-	0	0
Ultra Gel	37	96	24	65%	20	-	-	-
Squeezy	28	100	25	89%	120	40	0	0
Pocket Rocket	37	100	25	67%	15	-	-	-
Carb Boom	41	107	27	66%	50	50	0	0
Hammer Gel	2 Tbsp (30ml)	91	23	77%	23	-	0	0

- Dash indicates value unknown

7 • Recipes

The following recipes are a compilation of some borrowed and some original recipes. The cookbooks mentioned have a great selection of other recipes to offer. Check them out at your local bookstore.

Quick and Easy Meal Ideas

1. Rockin' Moroccan Stew From Crazy Plates: Janet and Greta Podeleski, Granet Publishing
Moroccan vegetable stew with sweet potatoes, chickpeas and ginger in a yummy peanut sauce. This recipe is great served with warm bread. Leftovers are easy to pack as lunch and even freeze well.

2 tsp	olive oil
1 cup	chopped onions
1/2 cup	each diced celery and chopped green pepper
1 clove	garlic, minced
3 cups	vegetable broth
3 cups	peeled, cubed sweet potato
1 can (19oz)	tomatoes, drained and cut up
1 can (19oz)	chickpeas, drained and rinsed
1 Tbs	lemon juice
2 tsp	grated gingerroot
1 tsp each	ground cumin, curry powder, ground coriander and chilli powder
1/2 tsp	salt
1/4 tsp	pepper
1/4 cup	raisins
2 Tbs each	light peanut butter and chopped fresh cilantro (optional)

- Heat oil in a large, non-stick saucepan over medium high heat. Add onions, celery, green pepper and garlic. Cook and stir until vegetables begin to soften, about 3 minutes.
- Add all remaining ingredients, except raisins, peanut butter and cilantro. Bring to a boil. Reduce heat and simmer, covered for 20 minutes.
- Stir in raisins, peanut butter and cilantro(optional). Mix well. Simmer for 5 more minutes. Serve hot.

Makes 6 servings: **Each serving: 251 cals, 5.1g fat, 0.5 saturated fat, 8.9 protein, 45g carbohydrate, 4.3g fibre, 0mg cholesterol, 784mg sodium, % cal's from fat: 18%**

2. Grilled Chicken and Vegetable Bundles From More Choice Menus,

Marjorie Hollands, Margaret Howard. MacMillan Publishing.

What an easy and clean way to cook an entire meal in individual packages!

4	boneless skinless chicken breast halves (about 1lb/500g)
1 1/3 cups	(325mL) thinly sliced carrots (3 medium)
4	small zucchini, halves lengthwise and cut into 1-inch (2.5cm) pieces
16	small mushrooms, halves
1/2 (125mL)cup	chopped onion
1/3 cup	white wine or chicken broth
1 tbsp (15mL)	melted soft margarine or butter
1 tsp (5mL)	dried tarragon leaves (or 1tbsp/15mL chopped fresh)
1/5 tsp (1mL)	freshly ground pepper

- Cut 4 sheets of heavy-duty aluminum foil into squares twice as large as chicken breast. Spray foil with nonstick coating.
- Place chicken breast in centre of foil. Distribute carrots, zucchini, mushrooms and onion evenly over chicken.
- Combine wine, margarine, tarragon and pepper; spoon over vegetables. Tightly enclose chicken in foil by folding long ends of foil twice; lift short ends, bring together and fold twice.
- Grill bundles 5 inches (12cm) from barbecue coals for 45 minutes, turning occasionally OR bake in 350ºF (180ºC) oven until chicken is no longer pink inside and vegetables are tender. Makes 4 servings:

Each serving: 223 kcal (904kJ), 5g fat, 1g saturated fat, 29g protein, 13g carbohydrate, 4g fibre, 129mg sodium.

3. Low-Fat Fried Rice

This stove-top recipe is a basic idea that can be adjusted and varied to add some spice to your normal cuisine.

1 tbsp	oil
2	scallions with greens, chopped (or 1 small onion)
1 cup	sliced mushrooms
1	egg or 2 egg whites
2 cups	cooked rice (about 2/3 cup uncooked)
1 tbsp	soy sauce

Optional vegetables: broccoli, celery, snow peas, bok choy, Chinese cabbage, water chestnuts.

Optional protein: shrimp, beef, chicken, ground turkey, tofu, nuts, sesame seeds.

- Heat oil in a large skillet or wok over medium-high heat.
- Add scallions and mushrooms (and other vegetables and proteins, as desired); stir-fry 2-3 minutes.
- Push vegetables aside. Pour the egg into the skillet and scramble it.
- Stir in the rice, gently separating the grains. Add the soy sauce; stir thoroughly until heated. Makes 2 servings: *Per serving: 370 cals, 65g carb, 11g protein, 7gfat.*

Sodium Tip: The next four recipes are Campbell's Soup Recipes. They are fast, easy and tasty. The only drawback is that condensed soups tend to be high in sodium. Sodium content is often not a problem for athletes however individuals with high blood pressure should use prepared soups in moderation.

4. Beef Taco Bake Taken from Campbell's Recipes
Save time by purchasing pre-shredded cheese – you'll need a 4-oz package for the 1 cup shredded cheese in this recipe.

1 lb (454g)	extra lean ground beef
1 can (10oz fl/284mL)	Campbell's Condensed Tomato soup
1 cup (250mL)	Pace Thich & Chunky Salsa
1/2 cup (125mL)	milk

6 flour tortillas or 8 corn tortillas (6" to 8"), cut into 1" pieces
1 cup (250mL) shredded lower fat Cheddar cheese

- In a skillet, over medium-high heat, cook beef until browned, stirring to separate meat. Pour off fat.
- Add soup, salsa, milk, tortillas, and half the cheese. Spoon into 8-cup (2 L) shallow baking dish. Cover.
- Bake at 400ºF (200ºC) for 30 minutes or until hot. Sprinkle with remaining cheese. Makes 4 main-dish servings: *Each serving of 1 1/2 cup (375mL): 633 cal, 40g protein, 25g fat, 62g carbohydrates.*

5. Creamy Chicken Stir-Fry Taken from Campbell's Recipes
For variety, try different vegetables: snow peas, mushrooms, celery or asparagus.

Vegetable cooking spray

3 cups (750mL)	cut up vegetables (broccoli flowerets, sliced carrots and green or red pepper strips)
1 lb (454g)	skinless, boneless chicken breasts, cut into strips

1 can (10 oz fl/284mL)	Campbells' Condensed half fat cream of chicken soup
1/4 cup (50mL)	water
1 tbsp (15mL)	soy sauce
4 cups (1L)	hot cooked rice, cooked without margarine or salt

- Spray skillet with cooking spray and heat over medium heat 1 min. Add vegetables and stir-fry until tender-crisp. Set vegetables aside.
- Remove pan from heat. Spray with cooking spray. Add chicken in 2 batches and stir-fry over medium-high heat until browned. Set chicken aside.
- Add soup, water and soy sauce. Heat to a boil. Return vegetables and chicken to pan. Heat through. Serve over rice. Makes 4 main-dish servings: *Each serving 2 cups (500mL): 401 cal, 35g protein, 4g fat, 57g carbohydrates.*

6. Tuna Noodle Casserole Taken from Campbell's Recipes
For variety try a different type of pasta like spiral, penne or shell pasta.

2 1/2 cups (625mL)	dry medium noodles
1 cup (250mL)	frozen peas
1 can (10 oz fl/284mL)	Campbell's Condensed Half Fat Cream of Celery soup
1/2 cup (125mL)	2% milk
1 can (6.5 oz/184g)	tuna, drained and flaked
1 cup (250mL)	shredded lower fat Cheddar cheese
Paprika	

- Prepare noodles according to package directions. Add peas for last 5 minutes of cooking time. Drain.
- In 8-cup (2L) casserole, combine soup, milk, tuna and half of cheese. Stir in noodles and peas. Top with remaining cheese. Sprinkle with paprika.
- Bake at 400ºF (200ºC) for 20-25 minutes or until bubbling and hot.

Makes 4 main-dish servings: *For each 2 cup (500mL) serving: 542 cal, 35g protein, 12g fat, 73g carbohydrates.*

7. Easy Chicken & Pasta Taken from Campbell's Recipes

This recipe only takes 5 minutes to prepare and then you have 25 minutes of cooking time to relax.

1 tbsp (15mL)	vegetable oil
1 lb (454g)	skinless, boneless chicken breast, cut up
1 can (10 oz fl/284mL)	Campbell's Condensed Half Fat Cream of Mushroom soup
2 1/4 cups (550mL)	water
1/2 tsp (2.5mL)	dried basil leaves, crushed
2 cups (500mL)	frozen vegetable combination (broccoli, cauliflower, carrots)
2 cups (500mL)	uncooked spiral pasta

Grated Parmesan cheese

- In skillet over medium-high heat, heat oil. Cook chicken in 2 batches until browned, stirring often. Set chicken aside.
- Add soup, water, basil and vegetables. Heat to a boil. Stir in pasta. Cook over medium heat 10 min., stirring often.
- Return chicken to pan. Cook 5 minutes or until pasta is done, stirring often. Sprinkle with cheese.

Makes 4 main-dish servings: *Each 2 cup (500mL) serving: 520 cal, 39g protein, 11g fat, 66g carbohydrates.*

8. Turkey Loaf

Something to spice up your turkey and a spin on a your regular meatloaf!

14 oz	lean ground turkey
2 cups	bread crumbs
1	egg
1/2	cup chopped onion
1 tsp	salt
1/2 tsp	pepper
1/2 tsp	sage
1/4 tsp	ginger

- Combine all ingredients well and place in a loaf pan.
- Bake turkey loaf at 375ºF (190ºC) until inside is no longer pink (approximately 1 hour).

Makes 6 servings: *Each serving: 255 cal, 7.5 g fat.*

9. Designer Pizzas From More Choice Menus, Marjorie Hollands, Margaret Howard, MacMillian Publishing

Make your own pizzas to please everyone. It's also faster than a speeding delivery car. See instructions for cooking at the end of the pizza types.

Vegetable & Cheese

3/4 cup (175mL)	crushed and drained canned tomatoes
1/2 cup (125mL)	sliced mushrooms
1/4 cup (50mL)	cooked broccoli florets
1/2 cup (50mL)	chopped sweet green peppers
1/2 cup (50mL)	diced zucchini
2 tbsp (25mL)	chopped onions
1 tbsp (15mL)	chopped fresh or dried basil
1	crushed clove garlic
50g	crumbled chevre cheese
1 cup (250mL)	shredded light mozzarella cheese
1 tbsp (15mL)	pine nuts or slivered almonds

Each serving: 410 kcal, 12g total fat, 4g saturated fat, 22g protein, 54g carbohydrate, 5g fibre, 725mg sodium.

Greek Pizza

3/4 cup (175mL)	pizza tomato sauce
1/4 cup (50mL)	sliced black olives
2	medium tomatoes, thinly sliced
1 cup (250mL)	crumbled feta cheese
1/4 cup (50mL)	freshly grated Parmesan cheese
1/2 tsp (2mL)	dried oregano
1	minced clove garlic

Each serving: 411 kcal, 13g total fat, 6g saturated fat, 18g protein, 56g carbohydrate, 5g fibre, 1209mg sodium.

Ham & Pineapple Pizza

1 can (10 oz/384mL)	stewed tomatoes, drained
3/4 cup (175mL)	diced lean ham
1/2 cup (125mL)	drained pineapple tidbits
1/4 cup (50mL)	chopped sweet green pepper
1/2 tsp (2mL)	dried oregano
1/2 tsp (2mL)	dried basil
1 cup (250mL)	shredded light Swiss cheese

Each serving: 393kcal, 9g total fat, 4g saturated fat, 23g protein, 56g carbohydrate, 4g fibre, 954mg sodium.

- Purchase a plain gourmet Italian-style flatbread (14oz/400g).
- Choose one of the designer recipes.
- Bake each pizza on a baking sheet in 375ºF (190ºC) oven for 12-15 minutes or until heated and cheese is melted.
- Or, make individual pizzas, using smaller (100g) shells with 1/4 topping ingredients.
- Any of the tomato sauces are interchangeable and each is high in fibre, as well.

10. Personal Foil Dinners
Use what you have on hand – Minimal Clean Up – Fast and Tasty!

Use ingredients you have on hand....

Protein	Veggies	Sauce
Chicken breast, sliced	Carrots, green beans	Chicken broth, Italian seasoning Or Peanut sauce
Fish, cut into chunks	Carrots, zucchini	Zesty Italian dressing
Diced ham	Pineapple tidbits, peppers	Chicken broth, Dijon Mustard
Meatless: diced firm tofu,	Mushrooms, peppers, carrots, zucchini	Vegetable broth or zesty Italian dressing

- Fold a long piece of foil in half lengthwise. Double fold the two opposite sides.
- Spoon 1/3 cup minute rice, meat, a handful of veggies and 1/3 cup sauce into foil. Double fold the remaining edge.
- Place parcel on baking sheet and bake at 450ºF for 15 minutes.

Salads and Side Dishes

11. Chickpea Salad

For variation try adding any of the following: carrots, sesame seeds, parsley, cumin, broccoli or even a can tuna instead of the chickpeas.

2 cups (500mL)	chickpeas – drained
1 cup (250mL)	corn niblets – drained
1/2 - 1	green pepper chopped
1 tbsp (15mL)	Light Italian dressing
1	green onion stalk, chopped
1/4 cup (50mL)	vinegar (balsamic, white, cider..)
1/2 tsp (5-10mL)	mustard
Pepper to taste.	

Mix ingredients and enjoy!! *Makes 3 servings:* **Each 1 cup serving: 260 cals, 4g fat, 6g fibre.**

12. Three Bean Salad

Save time by making this ahead of time at night and bringing it in your lunch the next day!

1 can green beans – drained
1 can yellow wax beans – drained
1 can dark kidney beans – drained
1/2 - 1   green pepper, chopped
1 small white onion, chopped finely

1/2 cup (125mL)	vinegar – your choice
1/4 - 2/3 cup (50mL-175mL)	sugar
1/8 – 1/4 cup (25mL – 50mL)	salad oil

• Mix ingredients and enjoy!

13. Broccoli Cheese Potato From Mary Ellen McDonald, RD

Potatoes contain complex carbohydrates and supply protein and ample vitamins; they are delicious when dressed up with broccoli and cheese.

4 hot, baked potatoes

2 1/2 cups (625mL)	non-fat cottage cheese
2 cups (500mL)	cooked broccoli florets
1/2 cup (125mL)	sliced green onion
4 tbsp (60mL)	non-fat grated mozzarella

- Cut baked potatoes in half lengthwise, remove pulp and combine with cottage cheese, broccoli and green onion. Place filling back into potato skins and top with mozzarella.
- Microwave for 2 minutes per potato or until filling is hot and cheese is melted over the top.

Makes 4 servings: *Each serving: 360 kcal, 0g fat, 29g protein, 61g carbohydrate, 9g fibre, 7g sugars, 15mg cholesterol.*

14. Low Fat Home Fries

This is a great way to get your "fry fix" without the added fat.

	4 small unpeeled potatoes (Russet potatoes work well)
1 tsp (5mL)	dried onion flakes
1/2 tsp (2mL)	dried oregano
1/4 tsp (1mL)	garlic salt
	Paprika
1/2 tsp	chilli powder or tex mex spices
	Freshly ground pepper
1 tbsp (15mL)	olive oil or canola oil

- Preheat oven to 375ºF. Line a baking sheet with foil. Spray foil with vegetable cooking spray. Set aside
- Scrub potatoes; pat dry with paper towels. Cut each potato in half lengthwise. Cut each half into 4 long wedges. Set aside.
- In a small bowl, combine onion flakes, oregano, garlic salt, paprika, and pepper. Mix well.
- Brush cut-sides of potato wedges with oil. Sprinkle cut-sides of wedges with spice mixture. Place potatoes, cut-sides down, on prepared baking sheet.
- Bake until undersides are golden brown, about 30 minutes. Using a large metal spatula, turn wedges. Bake until potatoes are golden and fork-tender, about 15-20 minutes. Place wedges in a serving dish. Serve immediately.

Serves 4: *Each serving: 132 cal, 4g fat, 2g protein, 24g carbohydrates, 141mg sodium.*

Shakes and Snack Mixes

15. Sunny Orange Shake Dieitians of Canada's Great Food Fast by Bev Callaghan RD and Lynn Roblin RD. Robert Rose Publishing (2000).

This smooth, calcium-rich shake only takes a few minutes to make, and you can drink it on the go!

3/4 cup (175mL)	vanilla-flavoured lower-fat yogurt
2 tbsp (25mL)	skim milk powder
1/2 cup	orange juice

Combine ingredients together in a blender and blend until smooth. Makes 1 1/4 cups (300mL) *Each shake: 278 kcal, 10.8g pro, 1.9g fat, 0.4g fibre, 51g carbs.*

16. Banana-Berry Wake-Up Shake Dieitians of Canada's Great Food Fast by Bev Callaghan RD and Lynn Roblin RD Robert Rose Publishing (2000).
Try using frozen bananas in this shake for a creamier texture.

1 banana	
1 cup (250mL)	fresh or frozen berries
1 cup (250mL)	milk or vanilla-flavoured soy beverage
3/4 cup (175mL)	lower-fat yogurt (vanilla, or other flavour to complement berries)

- In a blender liquefy fruit and a small amount of the milk. Add remaining milk and yogurt; blend until smooth. Makes 3 servings:
  Each shake: 234 kcal, 8.7g protein, 3.8g fat, 3.2g fibre, 43.8g carbs

17. Heidi's Portable Chocolate Recovery Shake

Use this tasty shake when you are on the go or on the road and don't have access to a fridge. The powder mix is easy to carry to a workout and the shake has the perfect balance of protein and carbohydrate for recovery after exercise.

3/4 cup	skim milk powder
2 Tablespoons	chocolate milk powder

Add powders to a clean dry bottle or container with a volume of at least 500ml. Shake powders to mix well. When ready to drink, add 2 cups (500ml) of cold water and shake. Makes one 500ml serving *Each serving: 278kcal, 50g carbohydrate, 18g protein, 0.2g fat*

Variation: For a creamsicle flavour, substitute 1 Tbs of "Tang" orange crystals and omit the 2 Tbs chocolate powder.

18. Crispix Nut Mix

You can use any type of cereal you choose in place of Crispix such as Chex, Cheerios, Shreddies or even bagel chips, melba toast pieces or pretzels.

1 tbsp (15mL)	Worcestershire sauce
1 tsp (5mL)	onion powder
1 tsp (5mL)	garlic powder
1 1/2 tsp (7mL)	salt
1 1/2 tsp (7mL)	sugar
3 tbsp (45mL)	water
3 cups (750mL)	Crispix cereal
1 cup	dry roasted peanuts

- In a large bowl, combine Worcestershire sauce, onion and garlic powder, salt, sugar and water. Mix in Crispix cereal and peanuts until covered with sauce. Spread onto nonstick cookie sheet(s). Keep the mixture one layer thick and keep the sides of the snacks from touching.
- Bake in an oven preheated to 250°F for 20 minutes, and let cool for 15 minutes before removing from cookie sheets. Store in a sealed container. Makes 3-1/2 cups.

19. Popcorn Munch From More Choice Menus, Marjorie Hollands, Margaret Howard, MacMillian Publishing

8 cups (2000mL)	air –popped popcorn (1/2 cup unpopped)
2 cups (500mL)	small shredded wheat cereal squares
1 1/4 cups (300mL)	broken slim pretzels
3 tbsp (45mL)	melted margarine or butter
2 tbsp (25mL)	grated parmesan cheese
1 tsp (5mL)	chilli powder
1/2 tsp (2mL) each	garlic powder and celery salt

- In a plastic bag, combine popcorn, cereal and pretzels.
- In a small bowl, stir together margarine, cheese, chilli powder, garlic powder and celery salt; pour over popped mixture in bag; shake well to distribute.
- Spread onto large baking pan. Bake in 275°F oven for about 35 minutes, or until golden brown and crispy. Cool before storing in airtight container or small sandwich bags. Makes 11 cups. *1 cup svg: 120 cal, 3g pro, 19g carb, 4g fat, 1g sat fat, 2g fibre, 307mg sodium.*

20. Tempting Trail Mix

This recipe is very tasty so may want to pre-portion out the servings to avoid over eating

1 cup	cereal (cheerios works well)
1 cup	roasted soy beans (look for <10g fat per 1/4 cup)
1 cup	raisins (any type)
1/2 cup	bran cereal (omit for pre-exercise snack)
1/2 cup	dried cranberries
1/2 cup	mini M&M's (optional)

Makes Sixteen 1/4 cup servings *Per 1/4 cup serving: 130 kcal, 5g protein, 20 g carbohydrate, 4 g fat (1 g sat fat), 4g fibre*

Appendix a •
Canada's Food Guide

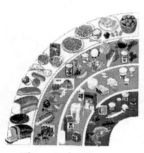

Main Messages From The Canada's Food Guide:
- Choose whole grain and enriched products more often.
- Choose dark green and orange vegetables and orange fruit more often.
- Choose lower-fat milk products more often.
- Choose leaner meats, poultry and fish, as well as dried peas, beans and lentils more often.
- Enjoy a variety of foods from each group every day.
- Choose lower-fat foods more often.

Serving Suggestions From the Four Food Groups:

1. Grain Products 5-12 SERVINGS PER DAY
2. Vegetables and Fruit 5-10 SERVINGS PER DAY
3. Milk Products 2-4 SERVINGS PER DAY
      Children 4-9 years: 2-3 servings/day
      Youth 10-16 years: 3-4 servings/day
      Adults: 2-4 servings/day
      Pregnant and Breast-feeding Women:3-4 servings/day
4. Meat and Alternatives 2-3 SERVINGS PER DAY

For more information or to print your own copy of the Canada's Food Guide visit the Health Canada Website at:
http://www.hc-sc.gc.ca/hppb/nutrition/pube/foodguid/index.html

a

Appendix b •
Balanced Snack Ideas

All of the following snack ideas have a combination of protein (underlined) and carbohydrate to provide you with lasting energy. Choose the portion that best satisfies your hunger. Get creative and make up some of your own combinations using the carbohydrate and protein ideas in Table 10 (p.82).

Quick snacks when you don't have access to a fridge
1/4 - 1/2 c	Trail mix (<u>nuts</u>, raisins, cereal, <u>seeds, soy nuts</u>...)
1 Tbs	<u>Peanut butter</u> with celery, or apple or rolled in a tortilla
2-4 Tbs	<u>Roasted soy nuts</u> and unsweetened applesauce or raisins
1-2 c	<u>Skim milk powder</u> shake (mix skim and chocolate powders, add water when ready)
1	Dried soup (look for brands <u>with 7-15 grams protein</u>)
1/2 - 1	<u>Powerbar</u> or other sport bar with 7-10g protein
1 pkg	Handi-snack crackers with <u>cheese or peanut butter</u>
1 can	Individual serving tuna with 4-5 crackers, pita or on salad

Quick snacks to grab from the fridge...
1	<u>Yogourt</u> (add granola or bran buds if you like a crunch)
1 oz/28g	<u>Cheese</u> (try pre-packaged cheese strings) and apple
1-2Tbs	Celery and <u>cheese spread</u>
1-2	Wraps: small wheat tortilla with <u>meat slice</u> and cheese slice
1 small	Burrito: tortilla, <u>refried beans</u>, light <u>cheese</u>, salsa (they freeze well)
2-4 Tbs	<u>Hummus</u> or <u>black bean</u> dip and veggies or 1/2 pita to dip
1/2 - 1cup	Three bean salad (<u>kidney beans</u>, green/wax beans, vinaigrette dressing)
1/4 - 1/2 c	<u>Brown beans</u> on 1 slice toast
2-4 Tbs	Each: salsa, light sour cream & <u>black beans</u>. Dip with baked chips
1/2 -1 cup	Potato salad with <u>egg</u>, lowfat mayonnaise and lowfat plain <u>yogourt</u>
1-2	<u>Egg (or egg white)</u> on toast, or <u>Deviled egg</u> and 1 cup of juice
1/4 - 1/2 c	<u>Cottage cheese</u> and fruit
1-2 cups	Salad with <u>cottage cheese or tuna or cheese or egg</u> on top.
10-15	<u>Shrimp</u> dipped in shrimp sauce
1-2 Tbs	<u>tuna or crab salad</u> on celery or 4-6 crackers

b

1-2	Spring rolls <u>with tofu</u> dipped in plum sauce
1-3	<u>Chicken strips or tofu</u> with "shake-in bake" dipped in plum sauce
2-3	<u>Meatballs</u> made with x-lean ground meat dipped in tomato sauce
1-2c	Soup: <u>pea, lentil, bean, chicken</u> or cream soup (made with milk)

Table 10: Carbohydrate and Protein Sources

Carbohydrate Sources *Choose whole grain for lasting energy*	*Protein Sources* *Choose lower fat options for heart health*
Grain Products • Whole grain bagel • Whole-wheat crackers • Whole-wheat bread • Multigrain cereal • Whole wheat english muffin • Popcorn • Multigrain flat bread • Pasta • Rice • Whole-wheat Pita • Oatmeal • Nutri-grain bar • Bulgar wheat	**Meat, Poultry, Fish** • Tuna packed in water • Lean deli meat • Low fat hot dog • Shellfish (shrimp, crab, lobster) • Roasted chicken/ turkey (1-3 oz.) • Lean beef (roast, ground) • Egg salad with light mayo • Boiled egg
Fruits • Fresh fruit • Fruit juice • Unsweetened Applesauce • Dried fruit	**Dairy Products** • Milk (skim, 1%) • Yogurt (0-2% MF) • Cottage cheese • Light cheese spread • Low fat cheese (<21% MF)
Vegetables • Chopped raw vegetables • Frozen mixed vegetables • Baked potato • Sweet potato • Tomato sauce	Vegetarian Proteins • Peanut butter, almond butter • Chick peas • Hummus • Brown beans • Black beans • Lentils • Roasted soy beans • Soy hot dog, soy slices • Soy milk/cheese
High Sugar Carbohydrates *Not suitable for lasting snacks*	*High Fat Protein Sources* *Use in moderation*
Granola bars Canned fruit in syrup Chocolate bars Jelly beans Gummy bears Liquorice	Regular cheese (22-40% MF) Milk (2% - homo) Nuts (almonds, peanuts, cashews...) Seeds (sunflower, sesame) Tuna packed in oil Cream cheese: not a good source of protein

Appendix c •
Sample High Carbohydrate Day

Approximate breakdown of 60-65% carbohydrate and 2500 calories

Time	Foods Eaten
7:00 am	Coffee, 1.5 cups Cereal, 1 cup Milk, 1 cup Water
10:00 am	10 Crackers, 1.5 oz Lowfat cheese
12:00 pm	1 Bagel, with 2 oz Sliced Meat, Lowfat Cheese Slice, Tomato 1 Apple, 2 cups Fruit Juice
3:00 pm	1 cup Yogurt 1/2 cup Granola 1 piece Fruit 2 cups Water
5-6:00 pm	Workout - 3 cups Water, 1 cup Trail Mix as a post workout snack
7:30 pm	1.5 cups Pasta with Tomato Sauce, 1 Chicken Breast, Tossed Salad with light dressing 2 cups Water
9:30 pm	1 cup Fruit, 1 Cookie 1 cup Decaf Tea

c

Appendix d •
A Specific Eating Plan For You

I Know What To Do But...

Eating right is not always as simple as "knowing what to do". Most of us know what areas of our eating habits need the most improvement however knowledge is only one piece of the puzzle. Changing habits takes commitment, new ideas and support. You may consider consulting a Registered Dietitian to help you put all the pieces of the puzzle together. Registered Dietitians are trusted professionals that will provide you with sound nutritional advice. A Sport Dietitian in particular will help you to

> **What is the Difference Between a Dietitian and Nutritionist?**
>
> **Dietitians are Registered Professionals. Similar to Doctors and Nurses, Dietitians belong to a legislating college that ensures they are providing safe and sound advice. In contrast, anyone can call themselves a Nutritionist. For nutrition advice you can trust, look for the RD, signifying Registered Dietitian.**

devise a specific eating plan personalized to your exercise schedule and your active lifestyle.

Here are some of the questions a Dietitian can help you answer:

Am I:
1. Eating the right quantity of food?
2. Getting the right balance of protein, carbohydrate and fats?
3. Deficient in any essential vitamins or minerals?
4. Getting enough fruits and vegetables?
5. Drinking enough and the right kinds of fluids?
6. Eating the right foods before, during and after exercise?

For a complete list of the services offered by Heidi Smith, Sport Dietitian refer to the website www.heidismithnutrition.com or call (519) 767 5011. To find another Sport Dietitian in your area try the "Find the Dietitian" search engine on the Dietitians of Canada Website www.dietitians.ca.

d

Appendix e •
Food Records

The following instructions and food records can be used for completion of a computerized dietary analysis. Many Dietitians will complete and interpret a computer analysis for you. Refer to Appendix d for information on how to access services from a Dietitian. You can also use food records simply to make yourself more aware of "what" you are eating, "when" you are eating and "how much" you are eating. Don't change your eating habits to look better than they usually are. Have fun with it and use the heightened awareness to fine tune your habits.

Instructions

1. Record all food and beverages, physical activity and important feelings. Refer to the sample food record to see the format suggested.
2. Measure your food to keep diet records accurate.
   - Use cup measures or teaspoon/tablespoons. eg: Put butter or margarine into a tablespoon, then scoop out to cover bread. Put cooked pasta into a cup measure...
   - For foods that can't be measured easily, read food labels to estimate quantity by weight. eg: If you ate 1/2 a 200g package of lunch meat, write 100g in the amount column.
   - **A quick guide to estimate quantity is your hand: Fist = 1 cup, Palm of hand = 3oz meat, Thumb = Tablespoon.**
3. For combined foods include a description of ingredients ie: Stir fry portion – 1 chicken breast, 1 cup veggies (onion, peppers, carrots), 1/4 tsp oil.
4. Use the "notes" column to record any **important feelings** (ie: overfull, headache, felt stressed, felt depressed). Include **additional product information** if available (ie: 2 cookies - 120 calories, 8g fat).
5. Enter the time and description of any **physical activity**. Ie: walking, biking, mowing lawn, heavy housework, going to the gym, any exercise including duration and intensity (easy, moderate, hard).

e

Tips to improve accuracy:
- Carry food records wherever you go, and write down as you eat.
- For an computer analysis: include food label information if available.
- Indicate any sauces or oils used in cooking.
- Keep a measuring cup and tsp/Tbs on your counter as a reminder.
- To estimate quantities when eating out, ask for sauces "on the side"

Sample Food and Activity Record

Below is an EXAMPLE of how to keep accurate records. Separate each component of a meal on to separate lines. Include a detailed description and amounts for each item. Remember to record water, exercise and notes on how you felt each day.

TIME	AMOUNT	DESCRIPTION	NOTES
8am	Large	Coffee, Tim Horton's	Tired
	1 Tbs	Cream	
	2 tsp	Sugar	
11 am	2 slices	Bread, whole wheat, toasted	only ate 3/4of it
	2 oz.	Tuna, light, packed in water	
	1 tbsp	Mayo, Hellman's	
	1 leaf	Lettuce, Iceburg	
	1 tsp.	Becel Light Margarine	
11:30pm	2 cups	water, tap	drank over 1 hour
2 pm	1/2 cup	Spaghetti noodles, boiled with salt	Felt satisfied
	1/4 cup	Spaghetti sauce, Prego's meat sauce	
	1 tbsp.	Parmesan cheese, grated	
3:30pm		Walked home, easy, 30 minutes	
4pm	1 large	Muffin, carrot and nut, home baked	had headache before
4:30-5:30		45 MINUTE RUN moderate 8km	
		Drank 1 cup of water during in my stomach	muffin felt heavy
8:30pm	4 oz.	Hamburger, barbequed	starving, ate too fast
	1	Hamburger Bun, sesame seed	
	1/2 cup	Lettuce, iceburg	
	2 slices	Tomato, raw	
	1 slice	Onion, raw	
	2 tsp.	Ketchup, Heinz	45 kcal per tsp.
	2 cup	Chocolate ice cream	Too full, Felt guilty

DAILY FOOD AND ACTIVITY RECORD

Name: _____ Date: _____ Day of the Week:_____

TIME	AMOUNT	DESCRIPTION	NOTES

Date of Birth(DD/MM/YY): _____ Height _____Weight_____

Appendix f •
Weight Log for Tracking Hydration

Use the following chart to track your fluid losses during exercise. Refer to Chapter 2 for a detailed description of hydration and performance. For an accurate pre and post-exercise weight, try to visit the bathroom first (if possible) and remove shoes, wet clothing, water bottle belts etc...

Date & Time	Weather	Workout	Fluids During	Weight Before	Weight After	Amt Lost	Recovery Fluids (lbs lost x 750ml)	Notes
May 11 8am	Cloudy, Cool (10°)	15km (96min)	500ml water	155 lbs	151 lbs	4 lbs	3 litres!	Next time bring two 500ml bottles

f

Nutrition For The Long Run

Date & Time	Weather	Workout	Fluids During	Weight Before	Weight After	Amt Lost	Recovery Fluids (lbs lost x 750ml)	Notes
May 11 8am	Cloudy, Cool (10°)	15km (96min)	500ml water	155 lbs	151 lbs	4 lbs	3 litres!	Next time bring two 500ml bottles

References

Chapter 1: Eating for Energy
1. Coggan AR, Coyle EF. Carbohydrate ingestion during prolonged exercise: effects on metabolism and performance. In: Holloszy JO, ed. Exerc Sports Sci Rev. Philadelphia, Pa: Williams & Wilkins; 1991;19;1-40.
2. Ivy JL, Lee MC, Brozinick JT Jr, Reed MJ. Muscle glycogen storage after different amounts of carbohydrate ingestion. J Appl Physiol. 1988;65:2018-2023.
3. Roy BD, Tarnopolsky MA, MacDougall JD, Fowles J, Yarasheski KE. Effect of glucose supplement timing on protein metabolism after resistance training. J Appl Physiol. 1997;82:1882-1888.

Chapter 2: Hydration
1. Briffa, J. Food for Health. Marshall Editions Developments Ltd. 1998.
2. J Sports Sci. v14 (#6); 497-502, 1996.
3. J of Sports Medicine, Volume 13, pgs. 399-406, 1992
4. http://www.gatorade.com/products_perform/thirst_quench/fluid_pyramid.html
5. Sport Nutrition Advisory Council (SNAC) binder
6. Graham et al, Journal of Applied Physiology, 85(3) 883-889, 1998
7. Position of Dietitians of Canada, the American Dietetic Association, and the American College of Sports Medicine: Nutrition and athletic performance, J Am Diet Assoc. 2000;100

Chapter 3: Achieving a Healthy Weight
1. Ross, Dagnone, Jones, Smith et al. Reduction in obesity and related co-morbid conditions after diet induced weight loss or exercise induced weight loss in men. Annals of internal medicine:, July 18, 2000. Vol 133(2):.92-103.
2. Am J Clin Nutr 1992 Mar;55(3):664-9

Chapter 4: Carbohydrate Loading
1. Roberts KM, Noble EG, Hayden DB, Taylor AW. Simple and complex carbohydrate-rich diets and muscle glycogen content of marathon runners. Eur J Appl Physiol Occup Physiol 1988;57:70-4.
2. Hawley JA, Schabort EJ, Noakes TD, Dennis SC. Carbohydrate-loading and exercise performance. An update. Sports Med 1997;24:73-81.

ref

3. Burke LM, Cox GR, Culmmings NK, Desbrow B. Guidelines for daily carbohydrate intake: do athletes achieve them? Sports Med 2001;31:267-99.

4. NISMAT Sports Nutrition Corner: Carbohydrate. (2000). Available: http://www.nismat.org/nutricor/carbohydrate.html

5. Kreitzman SN, Coxon AY, Szaz KF. Glycogen storage: illusions of easy weight loss, excessive weight regain, and distortions in estimates of body composition. Am J Clin Nutr 1992;56(1 Suppl):292S-293S.

6. Houtkooper L. Food selection for endurance sports. Med Sci Sports Exerc 1992;24(9 Suppl):S349-59.

7. J of Sports Medicine, Volume 13, pgs. 399-406, 1992